Basic Guide to
Dental Sedation Nursing

BASIC GUIDE TO DENTAL SEDATION NURSING

Nicola Rogers

RDN, NEBDN National Certificate in Dental Nursing, NEBDN Certificate in Dental Sedation Nursing, NEBDN Certificate in Dental Radiography, Tutor of the Year 2010 (DDU Educational Awards)
Dental Nurse Tutor
Pre and Post Registration Qualifications
Bristol Dental Hospital
Bristol
UK

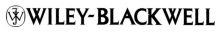

A John Wiley & Sons, Ltd., Publication

This edition first published 2011
© 2011 by Nicola Rogers

Wiley-Blackwell is an imprint of John Wiley & Sons, formed by the merger of Wiley's global
Scientific, Technical and Medical business with Blackwell Publishing.

Registered office: John Wiley & Sons, Ltd, The Atrium, Southern Gate, Chichester,
West Sussex, PO19 8SQ, UK

Editorial offices: 9600 Garsington Road, Oxford, OX4 2DQ, UK
The Atrium, Southern Gate, Chichester, West Sussex, PO19 8SQ, UK
2121 State Avenue, Ames, Iowa 50014-8300, USA

For details of our global editorial offices, for customer services and for information about how to
apply for permission to reuse the copyright material in this book please see our website at
www.wiley.com/wiley-blackwell.

Library of Congress Cataloging-in-Publication Data

Rogers, Nicola, 1962–
   Basic guide to dental sedation nursing / Nicola Rogers.
       p. ; cm.
   Includes bibliographical references and index.
   ISBN 978-1-4443-3470-8 (pbk. : alk. paper)   1. Anesthesia in dentistry.   I. Title.
   [DNLM: 1. Anesthesia, Dental–nursing.   2. Conscious Sedation–nursing.   3. Anesthesia,
Dental–contraindications.   4. Conscious Sedation–contraindications.   5. Dental Assistants.
6. Emergency Treatment–nursing.   WO 460]
   RK510.R676   2011
   617.9′676–dc22

                                                                        2011008574

A catalogue record for this book is available from the British Library.

This book is published in the following electronic formats: ePDF 9781444342420; Wiley Online
Library 9781444342451; ePub 9781444342437; Mobi 9781444342444

Set in 10/12.5 pt Sabon by Aptara® Inc., New Delhi, India
Printed and bound in Malaysia by Vivar Printing Sdn Bhd

1   2011

Contents

How to use this book

This book is a basic guide to dental sedation nursing, which has been written with dental nurses in mind. However, it could be used by other members of the dental team as it is a self-explanatory resource.

It has been compiled in order that any dental nurse, whether working within a dental practice that provides sedation or not, after reading would have a clear understanding of the roles and responsibilities of the dental nurse, enabling them to recognise good practice. It can also be used in conjunction with any course material that may be provided to dental nurses who are sitting the National Examining Board for Dental Nurses' National Certificate in Dental Sedation Nursing examination, as it has been written in a user-friendly manner covering all aspects relevant to the examination.

There is no intention of instructing/criticising clinicians, anaesthetists or any professionals on their role in the surgery, which have only been explained to further the knowledge of dental nurses. Any offence is entirely unintended and apologies are tendered for any perceived affront.

Dental nurses are subsequently reminded/warned that on no account should they undertake any duty that is solely the province of the clinician/anaesthetist or any other professional.

Acknowledgements

To my husband David and son Sean, both of whom I am very proud of and grateful for the love, patience and support they have shown while I have been writing this book.

To my parents and Valerie for always teaching me to reach for my dreams and for the valuable time they invested in me, especially my father, who has constantly given his time to reading and helping me correct the chapters.

To Chris Bell, my sedation course tutor, whose knowledge and skills passed to myself have made this book possible.

Photographs by David Rogers, ably assisted by Tina Huckle, Zara Plumley and Maria Tregale, courtesy of Southmead Health Centre, Bristol and Bristol Dental Hospital.

Thanks are also tendered to Wiley-Blackwell for permission to use various diagrams, partial texts, etc., and also to the General Dental Council.

Chapter 1

Introduction

LEARNING OUTCOMES

At the end of this chapter you should have a clear understanding of:

- Why dental sedation is used.

A small percentage of the population in any country actively avoids attending a dentist because of fear and those who do attend declare themselves anxious in a dental environment. The two main reasons for non-attendance are fear and associated costs. Patients who do not attend because of fear can be classified as being phobic, whereas others can be termed anxious. Other reasons for non-attendance can be attributed to lack of dentists in the area, difficulty in registering with a dentist or inability to access a dentist because of factors such as mobility problems. The provision of sedation in oral, intravenous, inhalation and transmucosal (off-licence) forms helps to overcome a patient's fears and anxieties, but not necessarily their phobia. However, by accepting sedation patients are able to undergo the dental care required to maintain a healthy mouth. These forms of sedation are explained in detail in Chapter 5 [1].

DEFINITION OF CONSCIOUS SEDATION

Conscious sedation is defined as 'a technique in which the use of a drug or drugs produces a state of depression of the central nervous system enabling treatment to be carried out, but during which verbal contact with the patient is maintained throughout the period of sedation. The drugs and techniques used to provide conscious sedation for dental treatment should carry a margin of safety wide enough to render loss of consciousness unlikely'. This means that patients must remain conscious and are able to understand and respond to any requests, (i.e. if the patient is asked to take a few deep breaths, he or she is able to do so). There is no such thing as deep sedation as any loss of consciousness is classed as a general anaesthetic and compromises the patient's safety. This definition explains the state of conscious sedation but not how it should be achieved. However, it is widely recognised that clinicians use different techniques involving the administration of one or more drugs through different routes, all of which provide patients with safe sedation [2,3].

WHY DENTAL SEDATION IS USED

Humanitarian reasons

Sedation can help patients accept treatment who have treatment-related anxiety and phobia [1].

Anxiety and phobia

Anxiety is a state of unease that a person can often relate to because of the memories of whatever is causing them to feel anxious. This existing memory may be something that was experienced by the patient or it could be a translated experience from their family, friends or media. Very often the patient is able to explain and relate to the specific cause or occasion in their life that results in their anxiety when faced with a similar situation/experience. As anxiety is controllable to a degree, patients who are anxious will attend the dentist for treatment and with good patient management they undergo treatment, with or without the aid of sedation, depending upon their treatment plan. These patients are often found to have sweaty palms and an elevated heart rate, so monitoring their vital signs is very important to ensure their well-being. Most patients are worried or concerned when attending the dentist, while some are frightened. Feelings of fear are a major contributing factor to how elevated a person's anxiety level will be. Basic fears experienced by patients are based on the following factors:

- **Pain.** Nobody likes pain and patients can associate the dentist with it and think/feel that they will experience some pain during their treatment.
- **Fear of the unknown.** Not knowing what is going to happen allows a person's imagination to flourish. Patients who associate the dentist with discomfort may think that they will experience pain when receiving treatment.
- **Surrendering oneself into the total care of another.** This could possibly make a person feel helpless and dependent, making them feel trapped and not in control.

- **Bodily change and disfigurement.** Some dental treatments can lead to an irreversible change in the person's appearance. Patients may fear that it could alter their appearance drastically and they would not be happy with this.
- **Claustrophobia.** During treatment lots of instruments are used in the patient's mouth. Some patients find this intolerable and are concerned that an item could be lost in their airway or that their mouth may fill with debris, making it impossible for them to breathe.

Phobia is an abnormal, deep-rooted, long-lasting fear of something which rarely goes away, making it very difficult to manage and treat someone who experiences this in the surgery. It is very hard to overcome this condition or to alter the way the patient thinks and feels and in certain cases cognitive therapy may prove useful. The cause of phobia is usually deep rooted and is often initiated from a previous experience that the patient cannot recall, (i.e. something that happened at a very early age which is now embedded in their subconscious). The patient quite often cannot explain its origin or why they are phobic about a specific thing. They have no control over it. This category of patient may never visit the dentist or will only do so when they are in extreme pain. If they do, they very rarely return for follow-up treatment once they are pain free. It is only normal to feel anxious when attending the dentist and anxiety is a feeling which most people encounter. However, a small percentage of population is dental phobic, with the condition being more common amongst women. Dental phobia starts in childhood or during adolescence and can be associated with the fears felt by parents. The parents phobia/fears can be transferred to the child by observation and the way they respond and talk about the dentist. It may also be associated with the fear of blood, injury or hospitals, due to a personal experience. Some phobias can occur on their own without having a rational explanation for their presence. Patients who are classed as dental phobic particularly fear dental injections and the hand-piece. If treatment is possible, the patient reacts by tensing their muscles, expecting more pain than they actually experience during treatment. Research has shown that patients who are dental phobic may have the same level of pain tolerance as that of patients who are not dental phobic. However, if their pain threshold is lower, or even if their threshold is the same, they feel more pain. Naturally, patients' level of phobia can vary and affect them differently. Some dental phobics can cope with the unpleasant symptoms they feel at the thought of attending the dentist, whereas others would rather extract their own teeth and be in pain than visit a dentist. Unfortunately, some dental phobics also have a sensitive gag reflex. This action is normal and provides protection against swallowing objects or substances that may be dangerous. However, a hypersensitive gag reflex can be a problem, especially when it encompasses all sorts of other foreign objects, (i.e. aspirating tips and water from the hand-piece) in the mouth. This makes treatment difficult because of

INTRODUCTION

constant retching which affects the patient's cooperation and concern that they may choke. Patients who have a dental phobia can benefit from treatment with conscious sedation, as any form will reduce their anxiety and relax them. In the case of intravenous sedation, which has an anterograde amnesic effect, most patients will not remember their treatment despite being aware of it at the time. However, excellent patient management is essential with lots of tender loving care being provided. It must be recognised that dental-phobic patients will be poor attendees, while some may never accept treatment, even with the aid of conscious sedation. If they do, they will be very difficult to manage [1].

Physiological reasons

When a person experiences pain or anxiety, it can lead to their sympathetic nervous system overreacting, possibly resulting in hypertension or tachycardia etc. This can have an adverse effect on their myocardium, especially in the middle aged and patients with pre-existing hypertension and coronary artery disease, as it places additional strain on their heart, which could lead to an emergency situation. By providing a form of conscious sedation to this category of patient, it allows them to receive treatment without unnecessary strain being placed on their myocardium. The reason this occurs is attributed to whichever method of conscious sedation is used, as their mode of action on the body will relax the patient and reduce their anxiety. This causes their sympathetic nervous system to work normally with little or no reaction [1].

Complex dental treatment

Most patients attending the dentist will happily receive routine treatment without the aid of conscious sedation. However, on rare occasions they may require an unusual procedure such as minor oral surgery. This can be more stressful, more complex and may take longer than routine treatment. A form of conscious sedation can be offered at the treatment-planning stage, or the patient may request it. This makes their treatment easier to cope with and less stressful for them and the team [1].

BIBLIOGRAPHY

1. Bristol Dental Hospital course notes.
2. Department of Health, Conscious sedation in the provision of dental care, www.dh.gov.uk.
3. Department of Health, Guidelines for Conscious Sedation in the Provision of Dental Care. A Consultation Paper from the Standing Dental Advisory Committee, December 2002.

Chapter 2

Medico-legal aspects of dental sedation

LEARNING OUTCOMES

At the end of this chapter you should have a clear understanding of:

- The legislation associated with the provision of dental sedation.
- The importance of the consent process.

INTRODUCTION

Law and ethics within dentistry are very interesting, but dry, subjects that quite naturally go hand in hand. However, this aspect must be taken seriously in order to provide safe, effective treatment and to avoid patient complaints. The General Dental Council (GDC) regulates the practice of dentistry to protect patients. They publish various booklets (Figures 2.1a–f), one of which gives guidance on the principles of good practice. These booklets address legal and ethical issues that the dental team may face on a day-to-day basis, providing an overview of what is expected to prevent such issues occurring. A couple of paragraphs within the Standards for Dental Professionals booklet deal with conscious sedation, where the GDC state they support letters of advice from Chief Dental Officers, guidance and recommendations of two publications for the practice of dental sedation and that they expect the dental team to implement these when treating patients with sedation. These documents are:

- *A Conscious Decision* published in July 2000 by the Department of Health (DH), known as a review of the use of general anaesthesia and conscious sedation in primary dental care.

Basic Guide to Dental Sedation Nursing, First Edition. Nicola Rogers.
© 2011 Nicola Rogers. Published 2011 by Blackwell Publishing Ltd.

MEDICO-LEGAL ASPECTS OF DENTAL SEDATION

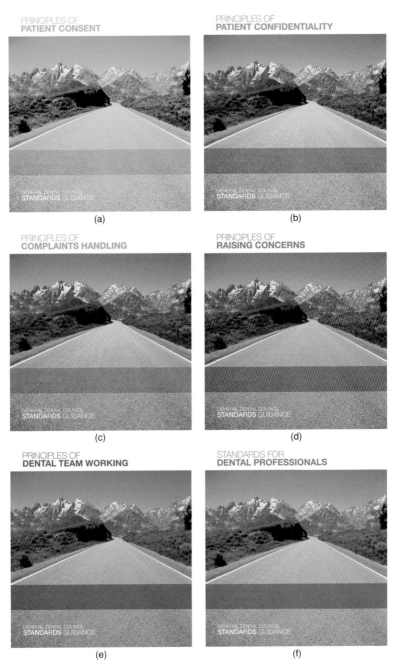

Figure 2.1 (a) General Dental Council's (GDC's) Principles of Patient Consent. (b) GDC's Principles of Patient Confidentiality. (c) GDC's Principles of Complaints Handling. (d) GDC's Principles of Raising Concerns. (e) GDC's Principles of Dental Team Working. (f) GDC's Standards for Dental Professionals. (Reproduced with kind permission from the General Dental Council. Information correct at the time of going to press. Please visit the GDC website to check for any changes since publication: www.gdc-uk.org.)

- *Conscious Sedation in the Provision of Dental Care* published in November 2003 by the Standing Dental Advisory Committee who are recognised experts within the field of dental sedation. This document was requested by DH [1,2].

RECOMMENDATIONS CURRENTLY IN PLACE WHEN PROVIDING DENTAL SEDATION

As pain and anxiety control are integral parts of dentistry, guidelines are in place for clinicians practising dental sedation techniques. These guidelines highlight the appropriate use of techniques and best practice reflecting the current definition of conscious sedation [1–3]. They state:

- The provision of sedation avoids a general anaesthetic for treatment of patients who have anxiety and/or phobia and for patients who are happy to attend but require a more complex procedure. The clinician will justify each provision of sedation, ensuring that the technique employed is relevant for the patient's medical, dental and social history and that the dental procedure to be undertaken will reduce the patient's anxiety levels without being too invasive. This is established by a thorough patient assessment with consent taken from the patient for the intended treatment. Ideally, only those patients who come under the American Society of Anaestheologists (ASA) I and II Medical Fitness Classification should be treated in the dental surgery (explained in Chapter 4). The clinician will, of course, know that the mainstay of pain and anxiety control is local anaesthesia and this must be the starting point before providing any sedation technique. They will also know that on occasions one sedation technique may not be successful and that they may have to adopt two techniques (i.e. a needle-phobic patient could be administered inhalation sedation to allow cannulation to take place). However, if the clinician chooses to adopt this approach, they would accordingly take into account the drug combination of the two [1–3].
- Most patients are suitable and conducive to intravenous, inhalation and oral sedation as adjuncts to aid them in the acceptance of treatment. The use of off-licence sedation in oral, intranasal and transmucosal forms is not recommended for routine use in the dental surgery. If practised, they will only be administered by a clinician in appropriate circumstances and setting [1–3].
- When a patient receives treatment with sedation, all members of the team must have undergone suitable practical and theoretical training, with every staff member in training being adequately supervised. Any training undertaken must encompass the drugs and equipment used, so that the team can recognise the difference between the normal and the abnormal. As a result

| Name: | | | |
| GDC Number: | | | |
Date Undertaken	Course or Activity Undertaken	Verifiable Hours	Non-Verifiable Hours

Figure 2.2 Continued professional development tracking document.

of training they will understand the action of each drug and also the use of the equipment. They will be able to clinically monitor patients, identify complications and know how to rectify them. The team must be capable of recognising and managing any emergency, so they must source training of this nature and undertake regular simulations. Training can be either through attendance at a formal course or in-house. Any person organising training for others must ensure that the training is delivered by appropriate instructors and in suitable settings. Continued professional development is vital to ensure that the practice of sedation is safe, relevant and up-to-date, with the frequency of any courses attended being variable, depending upon the area of work. All training received must be documented [1–3] (Figure 2.2).

- The surgery will, of course, be suitable for the provision of sedation, with both the treatment and recovery areas being spacious enough for the team to undertake treatment and manage an emergency should one occur with the chair's equipment allowing the head down tilt position [1–3].

- Should any complications occur the team must be able to respond accordingly and be aware of the associated risks. The entire team must be familiar with emergency procedures, having received training and updates on a regular basis. Simulations should be held within the practice. All emergency drugs must be available, restocked and kept secure, coupled with a means of administering them to patients. They should be checked on a daily basis to ensure that they are in date, with equipment serviced and maintained according to the manufacturer's guidelines. A means of securing a patent airway and administering oxygen must be available. Risk assessments must be undertaken in order to control the provision of sedation and to reduce the risk of accidents or mishaps. Dental practices should undertake audits to police the quality of care provided, ensuring best practice [1–3].

- For inhalation sedation, only dedicated machines for dental use should be used. They must conform to British Standards, be regularly serviced and cared for as per the manufacturer's guidelines, with records of all this being kept. The oxygen and nitrous oxide cylinders must be stored securely. For piped machines the colour-coded pipes must only fit into their respective outlets. They must also comply with the set standards and have fail-safe mechanisms installed so that the patient cannot receive a hypoxic mixture. Scavenging systems to remove the waste nitrous oxide from the atmosphere must be installed and used to prevent any health problems for the team. The nasal mask provided to the patient must be a good fit to avoid excess nitrous oxide being exhaled into the surgery [1–3].

- For intravenous sedation, the surgery must be stocked with all the required sedation and emergency equipment in order for it to be provided to patients, with all members of the team involved having sufficient and suitable knowledge and skills. All electrical equipment used must be calibrated, serviced and maintained according to the manufacturer's guidelines, with records of such being kept. Drugs and syringes must be labelled for correct identification and administration of any drug should be according to accepted current guidelines when titrated against the response of the patient [1–3].

- For oral sedation, the lowest possible dose should be prescribed, which is only sufficient to allow the patient to sleep the night before their appointment and to reduce their anxiety level. Patients must be advised that they will have to adhere to the same pre and post-operative restrictions as for intravenous sedation and they must be accompanied by a responsible escort. Oral sedation in this form is not to be mistaken for oral off-licence sedation. This specific technique, along with intranasal and transmucosal techniques, should only be undertaken in a suitable setting where the team have the knowledge and skills to provide this mode of sedation [1–3].

- To prepare patients for sedation, written and verbal pre and post-operative instructions must be provided to both the patient and their escort so that they both understand their respective roles before, during and after the appointment [1–3].

- Following treatment, patients must be supervised by an appropriate member of the team who will monitor and respond should an emergency arise, with all emergency drugs and equipment available. The recovery phase will initially commence in the dental chair until the patient is assessed as being ready to be moved to a recovery area, if available. The patient must be allowed time to recover and during this period the clinician must be available. It is not acceptable for any patient's recovery to take place in the waiting room. Not all patients recover at the same rate, with the rate dependent upon the drugs and amounts provided. Before being discharged, patients must be able to walk without help and be steady on their feet. They will be assessed for discharge by the clinician/sedationist and, when ready, discharged into the care of the responsible escort who will be in receipt of the post-operative instructions for both sedation and dental treatment. These instructions should also contain emergency telephone numbers [1–3].

- Excellent record keeping is important and must reflect the patient's treatment pathway and consent to treatment. Therefore they must contain the following details:
  - Patients' medical, dental and social history, including any previous treatments, general anaesthetic and/or conscious sedation and any change in the medical history/status.
  - Details of the assessment appointment.
  - The mode of sedation and the treatment being provided, the justification for its use and any patient preferences.
  - Written consent and that verbal and written pre and post-operative instructions were provided. The patient is still happy to proceed with the planned treatment and they have adhered to all instructions. The responsible escort is in attendance and details of the mode of transport home.
  - Details of the treatment appointment.
  - All monitoring details, cannula site, drug used, batch number and expiry date, drug titrations and times administered.
  - The recovery information and that the patient was assessed for discharge.
  - Any complications and statements of how the patient responded to the mode of sedation used and/or reactions within the recovery phase [1–3].
- Any dentist referring patients for treatment with conscious sedation will have explored all other avenues of pain and anxiety control before doing so. They will also be confident that the establishment to which they are referring their patient is practising treatment with sedation that adheres to the guidelines [1–3].
- Clinical visual monitoring and where intravenous sedation is administered, it is mandatory to use electrical monitoring by using a pulse oximeter and blood pressure machine. The team providing sedation must be capable of monitoring a patient's colour, pulse, respiration, blood pressure, level of consciousness and anxiety, also ensuring that the patient maintains a patent airway [1–3].
- Some children may be uncooperative and difficult to manage so they may not always be suitable for conscious sedation. In that event a general anaesthetic may be considered as a treatment option. When sedation is provided to patients, the team must have sufficient knowledge and skills to assess the

patient, prepare them for treatment and provide the chosen technique in a suitable setting. When children are assessed for conscious sedation, it must be remembered that children are individuals and have different levels of maturity and understanding. For a child who will not accept dental treatment with local anaesthesia alone, inhalation sedation should be the first choice offered. Intravenous sedation is not ideal and if on a rare occasion it is used, then it will be administered by a clinician who specialises in paediatric sedation. To reduce discomfort for children when applying a local anaesthetic, a topical anaesthetic should be used, and if possible, it should also be applied on the cannulation site [1–3].

MEDICO-LEGAL CONSIDERATIONS WHEN PROVIDING DENTAL SEDATION

These considerations are no different from those that the team must consider on a day-to-day basis when providing treatment [1]. These are:

- Taking and recording a patient's consent
- Maintaining a patient's confidentiality
- Accusations of assault
- Negligence

The consent process

Consent is when one person gives another person permission to undertake something such as dental treatment. It is granted once the person consenting is aware of what is going to happen and it can be withdrawn at any time. Consent can be written, verbal or a compliant action. For most procedures within dentistry, it is the latter two as patients enter the surgery, open their mouths for a dental inspection and then agree verbally to undergo treatment. Obtaining consent from patients for dental treatment is good practice, with many clinicians routinely taking written consent for various dental procedures where complications may occur, such as the extraction of impacted wisdom teeth. There is no recommended form, but whichever one is used, it must contain both the patient's personal details and the practice details. It must be completed in ink, without abbreviations and signed by both parties involved, with the patient receiving a copy. Only a qualified clinician can obtain consent from the patient and when doing so it should be in a quiet, private area to preserve the patient's confidentiality, allowing them to ask questions. A dental nurse cannot take consent, but good practice would be to ensure it was in place prior to treatment. If the patient is to receive sedation, consent should ideally be taken during a separate assessment appointment. This allows a cooling-off period, giving the patient time to reflect and consent should never be taken under duress. Consent is not a one-off action but an ongoing process and it should be regularly checked and updated, especially if the course of treatment is lengthy and involves several appointments. When conscious sedation is provided, a patient's written consent must be obtained, especially with intravenous sedation, with all eventualities being discussed and recorded, allowing the patient to detail any treatments that they do not wish to undergo. This is because midazolam, the sedative drug used, produces anterograde amnesia, which means that the patient may not be able to remember anything after the induction of the drug, including any conversations held. Therefore, if the treatment plan requires a change (i.e. failed root canal therapy) while the patient is sedated, the appointment will have to be suspended, the patient recovered and an appointment made for another day. This fresh appointment would be to discuss their options and further consent, as they would not remember the conversation despite appearing to be alert. This would naturally be time consuming for both parties and inconvenient for some patients due to the arrangements they would have to make in order to be eligible to receive intravenous sedation. This is a mandatory process, because if the clinician undertakes a dental procedure, without consent, the patient can have cause to complain and possibly sue, as this may constitute assault. The written consent in situ would provide evidence of the agreement as it would detail the discussions held and the treatment to which the patient consented. Any treatment undertaken that was not documented could mean that the clinician was negligent and at fault [1–4].

Types of consent

Consent is classed as either of the following:

- **Expressed**. This is where the patient either verbally agrees or completes and signs a consent form to receive treatment [1].
- **Implied**. This is where the patient accepts treatment by a compliant action such as sitting in the dental chair and opening his/her mouth [1].

Reasons why consent is required

- **Patient education.** As the treatment plan is discussed in full they are aware of what is involved.
- **Maximise patient cooperation.** If a patient is aware of the treatment plan and has been given the opportunity to ask questions, they are more cooperative as they know what to expect. There are no hidden aspects for them to be concerned about, so they need not fear the unknown.

- **Improve clinician and patient communication.** The clinician will discuss the treatment plan with the patient so that he or she can decide whether to proceed or not. A rapport is then built and the patient would feel more able to approach the clinician at any stage.
- **Protect clinician from complaints, claims and charges.** If the patient has had their treatment plan explained in full and the process is recorded, then there can be no misunderstandings/misinterpretations, as documentary evidence will be available.

When consent is required

Consent is required for the following:

- All sedation techniques
- General anaesthetics
- Clinical examination
- Radiographs
- Photographs
- Treatment
- Student observations
- Research
- Possible keeping of body parts

Validity of consent

For consent to be valid, the patient:

- must be able to give consent – they must be able to understand and retain the information being provided, consider it and come to a decision themselves [1–4];
- must give their consent to treatment without feeling pressurised by anyone, so that it is given voluntarily [1–4];
- must be provided with adequate information – the clinician will discuss the following with a patient regarding treatment:
  - Proposed treatment they require, together with the mode of sedation being provided [1–4].
  - Advantages and disadvantages of any proposed treatment and the advantages and disadvantages of the mode of sedation [1–4].
  - Alternative treatments and other forms of sedation that could be provided [1–4].
  - Any risks associated with the treatment that are higher than 0.5% [1–4].
  - Timescale of the appointment and be able to make the necessary arrangements, to reflect the pre and post-operative instructions for the mode of sedation they are to receive.

- Cost of the treatment and associated costs for the provision of sedation [1–4].

The information a clinician offers will vary from one patient to another as they have to decide how detailed it should be. This allows a patient to make a decision regarding the proposed treatment and whether or not they wish to proceed. Tailoring the information to suit individual patients prevents them from making a biased or unbalanced decision due to not being in receipt of all the information, or indeed too much. Once a patient is in receipt of this information, they can consent to treatment, provided that the clinician deems them competent to do so. If a patient is considered not to have the mental capacity to consent, then any treatment provided would have to be in their best interest. Some patients do not want to know the details of their treatment and this should be recorded in their notes. As conscious sedation is a specialist area within dentistry, patients are referred for treatment to clinicians who specialise in this field (i.e. the local dental hospital). Therefore, it is imperative that the clinician undertaking the procedure takes consent, as it is their responsibility to do so and not that of the referring clinician [1–5].

Who can give consent

Always

- A competent adult can decide whether to accept or refuse any medical or dental treatment. Only they can make decisions on their own behalf regarding the treatment they wish to receive or refuse. Being competent means that the person understands the treatment they require and the implications of receiving or declining it [1,4–6].
- Persons between 16 and 18 years of age. When the clinician obtains consent from patients between 16 and 18, they, as with any patient, will establish if they are competent, and if not, consent will be sought from the person who has parental responsibility for them. All people of this age are classed as competent and able to consent unless it is known otherwise. Their confidentiality must not be breached unless there is cause for concern for their health. However, if a patient between 16 and 17 years of age refuses treatment, the person who holds parental responsibility can override that decision if a refusal is not in the patient's best interest [1,4–6].
- A legal guardian, appointed by a court, or by a parent taking parental responsibility for the child can give consent where a child is deemed not competent. However, any decisions made must be in the best interest of the child, and if they are not, they can be overruled by a court. In an emergency, where treatment would be vital to prevent a child being put at risk, treatment would proceed while waiting for parental consent. In this situation, they should consult with a colleague to determine what action would be in the best interest of the patient [1,4–6].

MEDICO-LEGAL ASPECTS OF DENTAL SEDATION

Sometimes

- Adults considered incompetent in other aspects of life may be able to consent to simple treatments but not complex procedures where detailed information is provided. This is because they may not be able to understand all of it and will not be able to rationalise or realise its significance in order to provide valid consent. In these circumstances, the clinician would undertake treatments that were in the patient's best interest. The clinician could possibly take advice from close relatives and friends or carers to determine their knowledge of any opinions the patient may have relating to the proposed treatment [1,4–6].

- Children under 16 years of age who the clinician deems as Gillick competent and has the maturity and capacity to understand, retain and make a decision on the basis of the facts presented and fully understand the implications of receiving or not receiving treatment. It is only the clinician who can make the assessment of the patient's capacity to consent, and when classed as Gillick competent the child can consent to treatment without the person who holds parental responsibility being informed or giving their permission. The law states that a person who holds parental responsibility for a minor does not have rights over them other than to ensure that they come to no harm, and therefore, cannot prevent them from receiving treatment. Gillick competency is normally only used in special or exceptional circumstances. As with persons between 16 and 18 years of age, their confidentiality must not be breached, which includes preventing the person who has parental responsibility accessing the minor's dental records without their consent unless there is cause for concern for their health. Good practice would be to include the person who has parental responsibility in any discussions and if this is not possible seek the minor's consent to inform them. However, if a child under 16 years of age refuses treatment, the person with parental responsibility can override that decision when a refusal is not in the patient's best interest, despite them being deemed Gillick competent [1,4–6].

Never

- The natural father if he is not married to the child's mother, unless his name is recorded on the child's birth certificate with the registration of the birth taking place before 1 December 2003. For a natural father in this situation to hold parental responsibility, they must either marry the mother of their child, make a parental agreement with her or obtain a court order.
- Friends and relatives cannot give consent to treatment for children, as they do not hold parental responsibility [1,4–6].

Confidentiality

Patients expect any information they provide to the team to be confidential, as they are putting their trust in them. Therefore, all members of the team have a legal and ethical responsibility to maintain confidentiality in all matters relating to the patient. They must not divulge anything relating to patients and ensure that all measures are taken to prevent any information being inadvertently disclosed. They must never provide details of a patient without their expressed consent and keep all patient information secure, so that no unauthorised person can access it. Patients may discuss sensitive issues with the clinician relevant to their treatment. Therefore, on receipt of such information it must only be used for the purpose for which it was given. Information relating to patients can only be disclosed in exceptional circumstances without seeking the patient's consent. For example:

- If it was of benefit to them (i.e. their health was at risk).
- In the interests of the general public.
- If it was considered that a serious crime was imminent.

If this course of action should become necessary, where possible the patient's consent should be sought and if not given, despite persuasive techniques, minimal information should be released. If any person(s) considering the release of information without the patient's consent is unsure, then advice should be taken before doing so. A court of law may request patient information without their consent, but only the necessary/sufficient should be provided. The person providing the information must be prepared to justify their action. Patients must be made aware that their information may be shared with other healthcare professionals, awarding them the privilege of consenting, explaining the rationale for doing so. If a patient dies, their information must still be treated as confidential [1–6].

Protection of patient information

Any information received must be treated as confidential unless permission is granted to share it. The member of the team in receipt of such information is responsible for maintaining its confidentiality – therefore, they must ensure that it is stored safely. If being forwarded, it must be done securely and when finished with it must be destroyed in an appropriate manner. Dental records must be stored away from other patients, the general public and other healthcare professionals who have no need to access them. When discussing any patient's case, the conversations should be held in private where the content cannot be overheard. Screen savers are important to mar computer screens when others enter the room, with computers being password protected. Sensitive telephone calls must be taken away from the reception area. Any telephone enquiries regarding information relating to another's appointments etc. or a patient calling up for any results of treatment should be politely refused, because confirmation of identity is impossible, and furthermore, a conversation would be difficult to verify at a later date as there would be no written documentation to support it [1–6].

Accusations of assault

Any treatment undertaken without a patient's consent is regarded as assault, and therefore, the clinician who undertook it could be liable and accountable for any implications arising from that action. Patients can make allegations of assault – therefore, clinicians must never be left alone with patients as it would be one word against another, irrespective of gender and the treatment provided. Serious accusations can occur when patients are left alone with a clinician who is providing treatment using intravenous sedation. This is because the drug used can alter the patient's perception of what is occurring. Some may have vivid dreams believing that such things really took place. They are, of course, more vulnerable than patients who are not being provided with midazolam, a sedative which relaxes them, reducing their anxiety and providing amnesic effects. If an accusation is made and the clinician has not been chaperoned by a second appropriate person when providing sedation, then the clinician would be unable to defend himself or herself [1].

Preventing allegations of assault

Consent is a must, whether in written or verbal format. If it is thought that the patient may make an allegation, the clinician must ensure that written consent is obtained. The clinician will never undertake any treatment unless the patient fully understands the treatment plan and is happy to proceed. The clinician must never be left alone with a patient, ensuring there is a witness, should an allegation of assault be made.

Negligence

For a clinician to be negligent, they will have acted outside the law and/or will have undertaken dental treatment that is not acceptable. All clinicians have a duty of care, to ensure that patients are treated safely, with a high standard of dentistry. When a patient is provided with sedation to receive treatment the clinician's duty of care extends to the patient's aftercare. Once assessed for discharge, the clinician will, of course, be confident that they will be properly cared for by the patient's escort, as documented in the pre and post-operative instructions, given verbally and in a written format [1].

Avoiding allegations of negligence

Communicating with patients effectively regarding their treatment is vital. To avoid any misunderstanding, patients must understand which treatments are to be undertaken and which are not. Obtaining written consent for the provision of treatment with sedation or when there are any associated risks is paramount, as this will provide documentary evidence of the discussions that took place and the agreed treatment. Contemporaneous record keeping of the dental notes is vital as their contents will provide a record of the patient's past, present and future treatment. They will contain any advice given and discussions held, indicating how motivated a patient is within their care and if they have chosen not to take given advice. Any and all patient concerns should be highlighted. The clinician should inform the patient if they are monitoring anything within their mouths, such as an early carious lesion or other pathology. Staff should be well trained and know their role within the team to ensure that they do not work outside their remit, only undertaking duties that they have been trained for and those they are competent to carry out with confidence. Staff should record any conversations they have held with the patient over the telephone immediately, with the summary being factual, as patients can request access to their notes. They should also record any cancelled or failed appointments and non-payment for treatment. Dental records should be kept for the recommended time so that they can be referenced, should a case of negligence be brought by a patient who is no longer registered at that surgery. A safe environment should be provided for all, with all equipment being serviced at recommended intervals [1].

BIBLIOGRAPHY

1. Dental Hospital Course notes.
2. General Dental Council Standards Guidance document, www.gdc-uk.org.
3. Department of Health, Conscious sedation in the provision of dental care. www. dh.gov.uk
4. www.wellsphere.com/aging-senior...a-competent-adult.../617663
5. www.gdc-uk.org; Principles of patient consent.
6. www.patient.co.uk; PatientPlus.

Chapter 3
Role of the dental nurse and equipment

LEARNING OUTCOMES

At the end of this chapter you should have a clear understanding of:

- The importance of the role of the second appropriate person during a patient's treatment when receiving any form of conscious sedation.
- The importance of clinical monitoring.
- The equipment used in the surgery.

INTRODUCTION

During any treatment that a patient receives the dental nurse must remain in the surgery and when any form of conscious sedation is used as an adjunct to allow patients to accept treatment it is imperative that a second appropriately trained person be present at all times. This is due to the extended role that a person has to undertake in caring for a patient during treatment. Whoever the second appropriate person is he or she must have received the proper training. In normal situations, the second appropriate person is a dental nurse, but in some clinical settings it could be another clinician. However, in some surgeries where they have numerous members of staff there could be the clinician, a nurse to assist with treatment and a nurse assigned to the conscious sedation aspect of the patient's appointment [1].

ROLE OF THE DENTAL NURSE

When a dental nurse is the second appropriate person in the surgery assisting with patients who are receiving any form of conscious sedation their role will

Basic Guide to Dental Sedation Nursing, First Edition. Nicola Rogers.
© 2011 Nicola Rogers. Published 2011 by Blackwell Publishing Ltd.

encompass a wide range of tasks. They will utilise many skills which have been acquired during the early stages of their basic training. The required additional knowledge and skills must have been attained by taking a recognised course in conscious sedation. Best practice and the usual pathway for a dental nurse is to take a course that leads to the National Examining Board for Dental Nurses qualification in dental sedation nursing. However, there are many very good short-term courses available through various training providers that do not lead to qualifications. Advanced training is important for the second appropriate person to help them understand their role within the team so that they do not work outside that remit and are able to recognise the areas of patient care for which they are responsible. In order for a patient to receive treatment with conscious sedation in a safe, relaxed and calm atmosphere, it is good practice for the team not only to work together on a regular basis but also to establish a routine, so that there is a good working relationship. Before a patient attends their appointment, it is important that the team prepare for their arrival so that every aspect runs as smoothly as possible. It is here that the dental nurse, acting as the second appropriate person, would start their duties and responsibilities within the patient's treatment care plan [1].

Role of the second appropriate person when a patient is receiving treatment with conscious sedation

The second appropriate person will start by preparing the surgery, ensuring that it is disinfected and identifying primary and secondary zones. They will also ensure that all instruments for the procedure are sterilised and all materials and medicaments are prepared. They will prepare the appropriate equipment to reflect the type of sedation the patient is to receive, along with all the equipment required to undertake the medical checks and monitoring equipment. They will collect the patient's dental notes and radiographs and ensure that a signed consent form has been completed. They will, at some stage, read the patient's notes, paying particular attention to the medical history to make themselves aware of the patient's medical status and be prepared for an emergency, should one arise. They will refer to any previous treatments that the patient has undergone with conscious sedation to establish if there were any complications experienced during the treatment and recovery stages. They will also be aware of the amount of sedation the patient received. Keeping good, contemporaneous notes is vital for the team's reference purposes. These notes provide a history of the patient's treatment with the use of conscious sedation and allow modifications to be made at future appointments reflecting any written comments. A very important role before any conscious sedation treatment takes place is to ensure that the medical emergency equipment is present and functional by checking the drug expiry dates, ensuring that the oxygen cylinder content is sufficient and that portable suction is present. If intravenous sedation is being administered, the reversal drug flumazenil must be available. If inhalation sedation is being administered, it is important to ensure that the machine is safe to use, the scavenging system is attached and that there is good ventilation within the surgery [1].

INTRAVENOUS SEDATION

Role of the second appropriate person before a patient receives treatment

Once the surgery is prepared to receive a patient, the second appropriate person can greet them, introduce themselves and take them into the surgery, or preferably into a separate room, in order to undertake the medical checks required to ensure that the patient is fit to undergo treatment using conscious sedation. Upon entering the room, they will ask the patient and the patient's escort to take a seat while taking care of the patient's belongings. They will have previously prepared a blood pressure machine, pulse oximeter (Figure 3.1), weighing scales, if required, and a method of documentation to record the patient's response to mandatory questions, ensuring that they have and will comply with the pre and post-operative instructions. Some dental practices formulate a pro-forma that they can use as documentation to record the patient's treatment pathway from start to finish, whereas other practices may record this information in the patient's notes. It is a good idea to request that the patient's

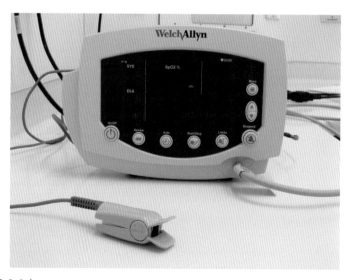

Figure 3.1 Pulse oximeter.

ROLE OF THE DENTAL NURSE AND EQUIPMENT

escort accompanies them at this stage so that it can be established whether after care for the patient will be adequate. This reinforces the importance of the role of the escort and the post-operative instructions that were provided at the assessment appointment. Once the patient and the escort are seated the second appropriate person should inform the patient that they will be looking after them during their treatment. They should commence by asking the patient the following questions:

- Are you normally fit and healthy?
- How do you feel today?
- Has your medical history changed since the assessment appointment?
- Has any of your medication changed since the assessment appointment?
- Have you recently visited the doctor?
- Have you any allergies?
- When did you last have any food or drink?
- Have you had any alcohol today?
- What arrangements have been made for you to travel home?
- Who will be looking after you at home?
- When are you planning to go back to work?

Once these questions have been answered and documented it is important to clarify with the patient's escort some of the answers given, in respect of after care. Record their name and take their mobile telephone number so that if they decide to leave the premises for the appointment duration they can be contacted. Once satisfied that the patient will be properly cared for at home the second

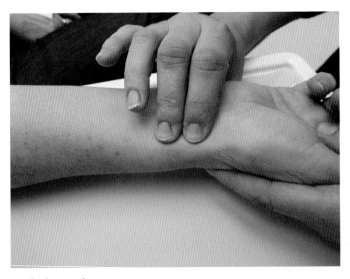

Figure 3.2 Pulse being taken.

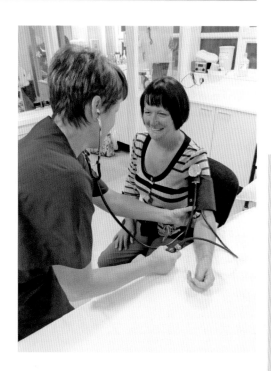

Figure 3.3 Blood pressure being taken.

appropriate person will take the patient's pulse rate (Figure 3.2), respiratory rate, blood pressure (Figure 3.3), oxygen percentage saturation levels (Figures 3.4a and b) and weight, if required, and document them. They will then present the readings to the clinician who will also act as the sedationist. It is useful to take the patient's pulse manually as this provides the rate per minute, the quality and strength of the pulse and whether it is irregular. This information is useful when monitoring a patient during treatment to identify any changes in the status and in particular when dealing with and diagnosing an emergency for comparison. They will note the colour of the patient's skin, their demeanour

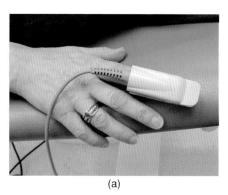

(a)

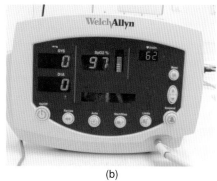

(b)

Figure 3.4 (a) Patient with pulse oximeter attached to finger. (b) Pulse oximeter monitor.

and whether they have false nails or are wearing nail varnish. If they are the varnish must be removed to prevent interference with the pulse oximeter readings or another site selected (i.e. a toe). Finally, the second appropriate person will ask the patient if they have any questions, answer them accordingly and if necessary explain the procedure for both the mode of sedation and the treatment being provided. A stop signal will also be arranged. Once this pre-assessment stage is complete, the second appropriate person will ask the escort to take a seat in the waiting room, advising them of the approximate length of treatment [1].

Role of the second appropriate person during patient treatment

The second appropriate person will ensure that the patient is seated comfortably in the dental chair and request their permission to apply personal protective equipment. They will, if necessary, introduce them to the clinician and wait attentively until the clinician is ready to commence. When all aspects of the appointment that the clinician wishes to discuss with the patient are complete, treatment will begin. Depending upon the sedation being used the role of the second appropriate person will differ slightly and this will be explained as the chapter progresses. For any sedation being provided the following role of the second appropriate person will apply:

- They will check whether a signed consent form is present.
- They will ensure that the patient has followed all pre-operative instructions relevant for the type of sedation they are to receive.
- They will act as a chaperone to both the patient and the clinician, irrespective of gender, so that if the patient had reason to believe that the clinician had acted inappropriately the second appropriate person will be able to vouch that this was not the case. Accusations can occasionally occur as the drug administered for intravenous sedation can lead to the patient experiencing dreams/hallucinations.
- They will aid the clinician in the clinical and electrical monitoring of a patient's vital signs, alert the clinician to any changes and respond accordingly. Monitoring should commence from the point the patient came into contact with the second appropriate person.
- They will assist with the procedure.
- They will reassure the patient throughout treatment.
- They will respond and assist the clinician in the event of an emergency.
- They will assist with the recovery of the patient. Some clinicians may decide to place this responsibility upon the second appropriate person. In this instance the clinician will remain on the premises.
- They will assist when assessing the patient for discharge.

- If the clinician decides that it is in order the second appropriate person may be requested to provide verbal post-operative instructions to the patient and escort, relevant to the mode of sedation received, the procedure undertaken and to furbish the patient and escort with written instructions for reinforcement.
- They may have to book a follow-up appointment.
- They will take the payment for the treatment and the method of sedation provided.
- Throughout the appointment they will practice excellent cross infection control, ensuring the health and safety of all, maintain the patient's diversity, dignity/rights and uphold the confidentiality of the patient.

Role of the second appropriate person while a patient is receiving treatment

Before the patient's treatment can commence they have to be prepared for cannulation. A simple explanation is given, advising them that its use is mandatory in order that the drug being used to sedate them can be administered. Discussions should be held with the patient as to whether they have any preference for the site of the cannula. The normal sites used are the antecubital fossa, the inner surface of the elbow or the back of the hand, known as the dorsum. They are advised that on insertion they will feel a small, sharp scratch and once inserted the cannula will be taped into place and tested to ensure that it has been correctly inserted by administering a solution (sodium chloride). Once successful cannulation is achieved the patient is told that the drug will then be administered. They will start to feel more relaxed and consequently less anxious.

Role of the second appropriate person during cannulation

The second appropriate person will have already prepared the following items for cannulation and administration of the sedation drug:

- **A tourniquet** (Figure 3.5). To restrict the venous return, thus engorging the vein so that cannulation can take place.
- **A disinfectant surface medi-wipe** (Figure 3.6). To cleanse the selected cannulation site. This must be allowed to dry prior to inserting the cannula, because medi-wipes contain alcohol which on insertion of the cannula will be taken into the vein and the patient will experience a stinging sensation. It is also not acceptable, once the cannulation site has been disinfected, for the area to be tapped to increase the engorgement of the vein as this would result in potential cross contamination and possible infection at the cannulation site. If this action is undertaken, then a new medi-wipe should be used.

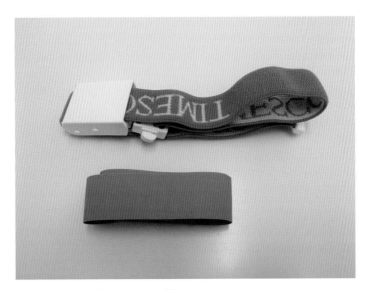

Figure 3.5 A non-disposable and disposable tourniquet.

- **A cannula, either a 22-gauge Venflon** (Figure 3.7), **a Y-can** (Figure 3.8) **or a 23-gauge butterfly needle** (Figure 3.9). To gain access into the vein, which, once sited, is known as an indwelling cannula in order to administer the drug. When placing a cannula the clinician will not probe, but be decisive. Probing can be very painful for the patient. Best and modern-day practice is to use a Venflon or a Y-can.

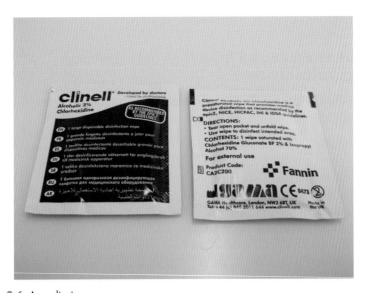

Figure 3.6 A medi-wipe.

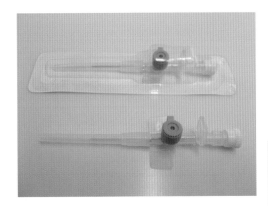

Figure 3.7 22-gauge Venflon.

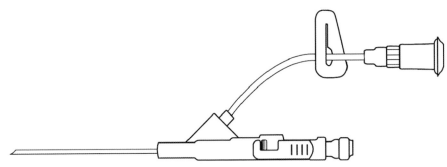

Figure 3.8 Y-can. (From Hollins, C. (2008) *Levison's Textbook for Dental Nurses,* 10th edn. Reproduced with permission from John Wiley & Sons.)

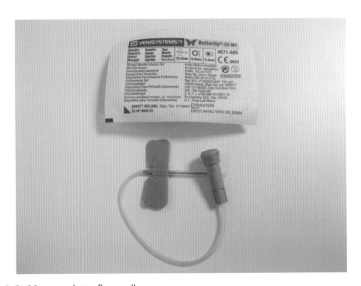

Figure 3.9 23-gauge butterfly needle.

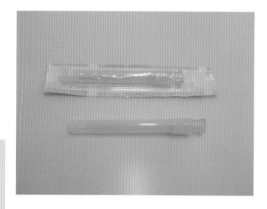

Figure 3.10 23-gauge drawing-up needle.

- **Two 23-gauge drawing-up needles** (Figure 3.10). One to draw the drug into a sterile syringe and the other to draw the flush into a sterile syringe. There are other available sizes of drawing-up needles, with the 23-gauge needle being the ideal choice as it is a filter needle, which means that it will filter any potential minute particles of glass that may have dropped into the glass ampoule. This prevents such particles from being drawn into the sterile syringe and being administered to the patient. The length of the needle means that it will reach the bottom of the glass ampoule drawing the entire drug into the syringe.
- **A 5ml sodium chloride flush** (Figure 3.11). To administer when the cannula is in place after ensuring that it has been sited properly. Sodium chloride is used, because it is compatible with the body. If cannulation has been unsuccessful it will not cause damage to the internal tissues as it disperses. Some clinicians may not use a flush after cannulation to check that it has been sited correctly. This means that as they administer the drug, given that cannulation has failed, the drug would disperse into the internal tissues. As a result, they have to estimate how much of the drug dispersed into the tissues and take this into account when titrating the remainder of the

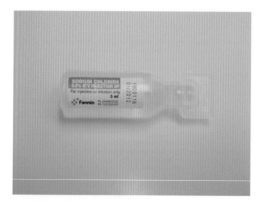

Figure 3.11 5ml sodium chloride flush.

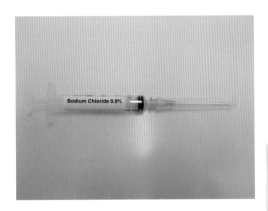

Figure 3.12 Sterile syringe with sodium chloride label.

drug, because the dispersed drug will eventually act upon the patient's body. If cannulation is unsuccessful it may be left in situ. This, of course, is at the clinician's discretion. Another cannula will be required and another site selected.

- **A 2ml sterile syringe with a sodium chloride label placed** (Figure 3.12). This is to contain the flush used to ensure that the cannula is sited correctly.
- **A 5ml sterile syringe with a drug label (midazolam) placed** (Figure 3.13). This is to contain the drug prior to administration.
- **The sedation drug to be used, midazolam** (Figure 3.14). To sedate the patient.

The second appropriate person will also have ensured that the reversal drug flumazenil is available, together with a 5ml sterile syringe and a 23-gauge drawing-up needle (Figure 3.15), which should be drawn up and administered to a patient only in the event of over sedation. This constitutes an emergency. The reversal drug must only be titrated to a patient during an emergency after all other basic assessments, airway management and the administration of oxygen have failed. It is not acceptable to use it as a means of reversing the action of the sedation drug, so that the patient can be discharged more quickly in order to shorten the appointment time.

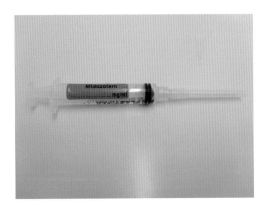

Figure 3.13 Sterile syringe with midazolam label.

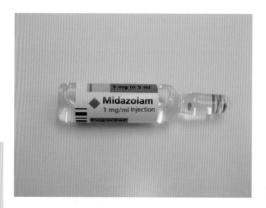

Figure 3.14 Ampoule of midazolam.

When a patient is having a cannula placed, the second appropriate person will undertake the following duties:

- They must ensure that the patient is seated comfortably and that the chair is placed in a high position, with the back semi-supine. This allows the drainage of blood into the cannulation site when the arm is lowered and in the event of a patient feeling faint they are already semi-supine.
- If required they will aid the clinician in locating a suitable vein to place the cannula and if the patient has cold hands they must provide a source of heat such as a jug of warm water. The cannulation will then be easier, as warm hands provide better visibility of the patient's veins, because they will engorge, as opposed to cold hands where the veins become more difficult to locate.
- They may have to pass the tourniquet to the clinician. Some clinicians may request that the second appropriate person applies a tourniquet (Figures 3.16 and 3.17). Some clinicians do not use tourniquets. Instead, they request that the second appropriate person places both hands around the patient's arm to apply pressure (Figure 3.18), thereby providing the same function as a tourniquet.

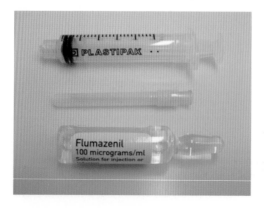

Figure 3.15 Ampoule of flumazenil, a 5ml syringe and a 23-gauge drawing-up needle.

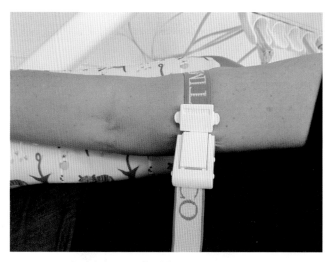

Figure 3.16 Tourniquet placed on antecubital fossa.

- Once the veins are engorged they will pass the medi-wipe to the clinician and when it has been used accept it in exchange for the cannula.
- When the cannula is being inserted (Figure 3.19) it is important that the patient is put at ease. The second appropriate person should talk to the patient and remind them that they will feel a sharp scratch as the cannula is being inserted. This is so that the patient does not jump on insertion. A back flash of blood will appear within the cannula giving an indication that it has

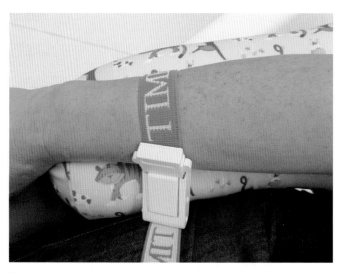

Figure 3.17 Tourniquet placed on lower arm.

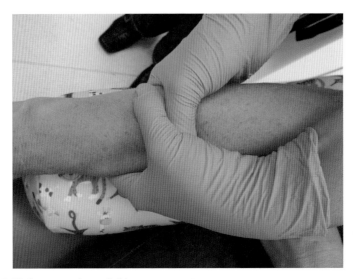

Figure 3.18 Lower arm being held to engorge vein.

been inserted into the vein (Figure 3.20). However, this indication is not a
guarantee of successful cannulation. The second appropriate person should
also make small talk to occupy the patient, taking their thoughts away from
the placement, as most patients find this part of their treatment unpleasant.
• Once the cannula has been inserted they may be requested to apply pressure
  at the point (Figure 3.21) of entry to restrict blood flow while the clinician

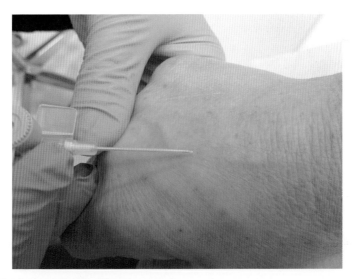

Figure 3.19 Placement of a 22-gauge cannula.

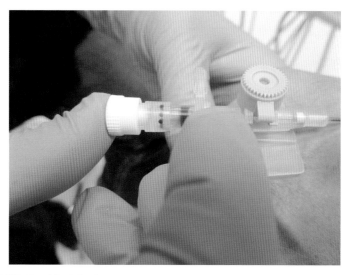

Figure 3.20 Blood flash back.

removes the introducing needle. The clinician will then remove the end cap, place it onto the cannula where the introducing needle was removed (Figure 3.22). This is known as the luer lock (Figure 3.23). Some clinicians request patients to raise their arm when removing the introducing needle in order to place the cap. This should prevent blood flow from the area.

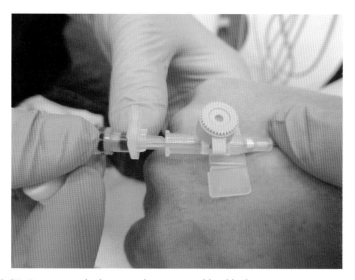

Figure 3.21 Pressure applied to cannula to prevent blood leakage.

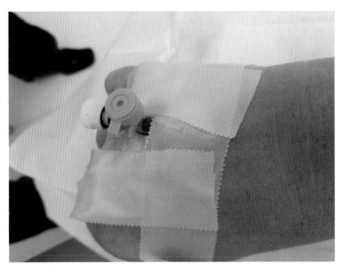

Figure 3.22 Cap placed onto luer lock.

- They must have a sharps bin (Figure 3.24) at hand for the clinician to place the used introducing needle.
- The second appropriate person may be requested to remove the tourniquet.
- The 2ml sterile labelled syringe, previously drawn up by the clinician, containing the sodium chloride flush will be passed to the clinician, stating the contents of the syringe. The batch number and the expiry date should have already been checked with the clinician and documented using the method of recording a patient's treatment pathway.

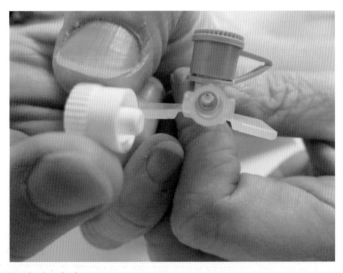

Figure 3.23 The luer lock.

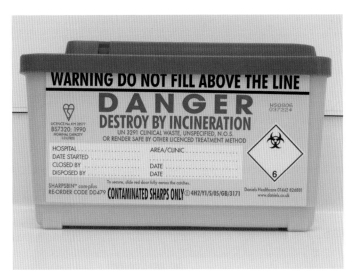

Figure 3.24 A sharps bin.

- As the sodium chloride flush is being administered the cannulation site should be observed ensuring its correct position. If swelling appears it will be an indication that the sodium chloride flush has dispersed into the surrounding tissues and that the cannula has pierced the vein wall. The raised area will look somewhat like a fried egg. The second appropriate person should inform the patient that they will experience a cold sensation travelling up their arm and that there should be no pain. Any failed cannulation must be recorded on/in the documentation of the patient's treatment pathway, along with the successful cannulation, recording the size of the cannula and the site used.
- Once it has been established that cannulation has been successful they will secure the cannula with either non-allergenic tape or a Venflon dressing, taking care not to pull the cannula out of the vein wall.
- They will place the pulse oximeter probe onto the patient's finger, explaining the reason for its use. They will have previously set the pulse and oxygen saturation level warning alarms that are incorporated in the pulse oximeter to suit the physiology of the patient.
- They will now pass the 5ml sterile, labelled syringe, containing the sedation drug to the clinician previously drawn up by him/her, stating its contents. Once again, the batch number and the expiry date should have been checked with the clinician and documented using the method of recording a patient's treatment pathway.
- When the sedation drug is titrated to the patient, against their response, the second appropriate person should continue talking to the patient, as their speech is a good indication of when the drug is taking effect. They will start to slur words, with their response to questions being slower. The second

appropriate person may be expected to advise the patient what they may experience and ask them how they are feeling. To establish if sedation is sufficient they may ask the patient to extend an arm and touch their nose. This action is known as the Eve sign. This tests the patient's coordination. If they can touch their nose they are classed as Eve sign negative and they are not adequately sedated. If they cannot find their nose or carry out the task slowly then they are Eve sign positive and are adequately sedated. Other factors need to be taken into account to establish whether the patient is adequately sedated. Observance of their general demeanour, their vital signs and level of consciousness or any adverse reactions must also be looked for. Continue to praise and reassure the patient.

- During the administration of the drug, they will record, once again using the method of documenting the patient's treatment, the initial bolus and any incremental titrations of the drug given. It is important to make a note of the time. The patient's percentage of saturated oxygen and pulse must also be recorded, along with a brief statement of the patient's response – for example, if the patient is still responsive – Eve sign negative – or if the patient is relaxed with slurred speech – Eve sign positive.

Once the patient is relaxed and cooperative, possibly sleepy but still conscious and the clinician deems them to be nicely sedated, the treatment can commence.

Role of the second appropriate person during the patient's treatment

The second appropriate person will assist in accordance with the treatment that the patient is receiving and, in addition, will perform the following tasks:

- They will continue to monitor the patient's vital signs by observing the patient's colour, demeanour and level of consciousness, paying particular attention to their respiratory rate as the drug used (midazolam) to sedate patients can cause respiratory depression. They should also periodically look at the pulse oximeter ensuring that the patient's percentage of saturated oxygen and pulse rate are still within the normal limits for that patient. It is useful to take a pulse manually for comparison with the initial recording at the assessment stage. The electrical equipment used is not to be relied upon as it is an aid to monitoring and not a substitute for clinical monitoring. Clinical judgement should be acted/relied upon should the occasion arise, as the pulse oximeter can provide abnormal readings. The alarms may sound due to sensitivity, attributed to various outside influences, which will be explained later in this chapter. In the event that the second appropriate person recognises any changes in the patient's level of consciousness or are unhappy about their vital signs, these concerns must be relayed to the clinician. The clinician will also monitor a patient's vital signs when providing treatment – however, they rely heavily on the second appropriate person as they are concentrating on the treatment being administered.

- They will constantly praise and reassure the patient throughout the period of treatment.
- They will document any further administration of drug titrated to the patient and if no further amounts are provided during treatment, record the patient's percentage of saturated oxygen and pulse rate every 15–20 minutes.
- In the event that the patient experiences an emergency or they become over-sedated, the second appropriate person would respond accordingly, assisting as directed by the clinician.
- They will record a brief overview of the patient's response to treatment with intravenous sedation.

Once treatment has been completed, the patient will need to be recovered prior to being discharged into the care of their escort. Encouraging the patient not to sleep and to expedite their recovery the dental chair is brought up very slowly to a sitting position. As the patients may have had their eyes closed during treatment, or have been sleeping, it is important to inform them of this so that they do not become alarmed.

Role of the second appropriate person during the patient's recovery period

Some establishments that provide intravenous sedation have a separate area for patient recovery. However, not all have the luxury of the space that will be required to provide this facility – therefore, the norm is for the patient to recover in the dental chair. Patients cannot be allowed to leave the dental surgery until 1 hour has elapsed since the last titration of drug was administered. As soon as the patient's face has been refreshed and all traces of treatment have been removed the second appropriate person will perform the following tasks:

- They will take all dental instruments to be sterilised and put away all materials, medicaments and equipment. They will ensure that all sharps are removed and all clinical waste is placed in the appropriate bins.
- They will ensure that all documentation relating to the sodium chloride flush and drug used is recorded before disposing of the empty ampoules into the sharps bin or container for waste drugs. If any drug or flush is left in the syringes, they will dispose of same by squirting the solution into the sharps bin before disposing of the syringe or by squirting it into a cotton wool ball/swab and place it into the sharps bin or the clinical waste. This may differ according to local protocol.
- They will document the time the treatment finished and the total amount of drug the patient received.

- On instruction from the clinician they will invite the escort into the surgery to sit with the patient and inform them how the treatment had progressed.
- They will reassure the patient, answering any questions that the patient and/or escort may have.
- They will continue to monitor the patient, documenting the percentage of saturated oxygen and pulse rate.
- They will take a post-operative blood pressure, if required.
- If requested by the clinician they will provide written and verbal post-operative instructions for the dental treatment and the sedation. This must include the telephone number of the dental surgery, so that if it becomes necessary, the patient or escort can make contact.
- They will assist in assessing or be requested by the clinician to assess the patient for discharge by taking the patient for a little walk establishing how steady they are on their feet. When undertaking this, it is important to ask the patient to place their feet firmly on the floor prior to standing and inform them that if at any stage they feel dizzy, light-headed or funny, they are to sit down and this assessment can be attempted later.
- Once the clinician is happy that the patient is fit for discharge, upon instruction/direction they will remove the cannula (Figure 3.25) and place it in the sharps bin, apply pressure to the site and document the time on/in the method of documenting the patient's treatment. The clinician may choose to remove the cannula personally – therefore, the second appropriate person will assist by providing a dressing and a sharps container. Patients should be kept for at least an hour after the last titration of drug before being discharged.
- They will assist the patient, with the help of the escort, to the car.

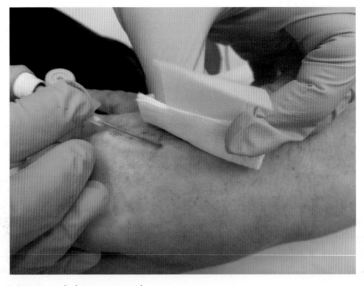

Figure 3.25 Cannula being removed.

- They will ensure that the method of documenting the patient's treatment is complete by adding the time the patient was discharged, coupled with a statement of how the patient responded while recovering.
- Once the patient has left the building the second appropriate person will carry out any unfinished cross infection control measures, tidy up and put away items not required while preparing the surgery for the next patient.

INHALATION SEDATION

Role of the second appropriate person when a patient is receiving treatment

Before a patient can receive treatment with inhalation sedation the surgery must be prepared. Ensure that there is good ventilation and that the machine being used, whether a mobile relative analgesia machine or a piped system, is checked, making sure that it is safe for use, as explained in Chapter 5. There should also be sufficient gases for the procedure. These checks are normally undertaken by the second appropriate person. It is vital that once undertaken these are recorded on the documentation used for the patient's treatment pathway, so that there is no confusion. This avoids any potential complications. The second appropriate person will also ensure that the scavenging system to be used is attached/functional and prepare a range of masks for use, bearing in mind that the patient may not have brought theirs [1].

Role of the second appropriate person before a patient receives treatment

Upon arrival of a patient who is expected to receive treatment with inhalation sedation the second appropriate person will perform the following tasks:

- They will greet the patient and start to monitor their vital signs.
- They will ask them and their escort, if they have been accompanied by one, to take a seat.
- They will ask the patient how they are feeling and whether they are suffering from a cold or have difficulty breathing through their nose, explaining that if they have the inhalation sedation will be ineffective. Consequently the appointment will have to be re-scheduled.
- They will check that the patient has followed all pre-operative instructions.
- They will ask the patient if they have brought the mask that they were provided with during the acclimatisation appointment.
- Depending upon the practice, they will take the patient's blood pressure, respiratory and pulse rates, recording them on/in the patient's method of documentation. Not all clinicians request these medical checks be under-taken for inhalation sedation, as the majority of patients treated are children

ROLE OF THE DENTAL NURSE AND EQUIPMENT

and these procedures can be uncomfortable for them, which can enhance nervousness.

- They will answer any questions that the patient or their escort may have.
- They will remind the patient what to expect and how they may feel during their treatment, providing a brief explanation, advising them that they will start to feel more relaxed, akin to floating/dreaming and they may experience some tingling in various parts of their body. They will also inform them that when they are settled in the dental chair the clinician will converse with them and invite them to put their mask on and the sedation will start to take effect [1].
- Once the patient has been prepared for treatment, they are shown into the surgery where everything required has been previously prepared and settled into the chair. The relative analgesia machine is already switched on with the gas mixture dial set at 100% oxygen.

Role of the second appropriate person during a patient's treatment

The second appropriate person will perform the following tasks:

- Give a brief explanation of the equipment to be used.
- Reassure and monitor the patient's vital signs.
- Help the patient to place the mask over their nose (Figure 3.26), ensure that it fits comfortably and is not too big, ensuring that there are no leaks. They will also ensure that the tubing to which the mask fits is secure and will hold the mask in place throughout treatment [1].

The clinician at this point will start to administer the oxygen by opening the flow meter, which will be set at approximately 8L/min for an adult and approximately 6L/min for a child. They will then slowly introduce the nitrous oxide, observing the patient's response, talk to them in a nice, calm, soft and hypnotic voice asking them to imagine they are doing something else or are somewhere else, to further relax them [1]. This makes them more conducive

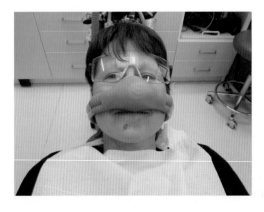

Figure 3.26 Mask placed on patient's nose.

ROLE OF THE DENTAL NURSE AND EQUIPMENT

to treatment. While the patient is being sedated the second appropriate person will perform the following tasks:

- They will continue to monitor the patient's vital signs ensuring that they are within the normal limits and the patient is not uncomfortable. As a pulse oximeter is not normally used clinical monitoring is very important to ensure that the patient doesn't become over sedated and suffers an emergency or an adverse reaction. Pulse oximeters are not utilised with inhalation sedation as the patient receives a minimum of 30% oxygen throughout their treatment. This minimal percentage is attributed to the inhalation sedation machine having this feature inbuilt. As this is more than in atmospheric air, all that would be indicated on the machine is that the patient has a high percentage of saturated oxygen available for their body requirements.
- They will record the time and the percentages of nitrous oxide and oxygen administered on/in the documentation used for the patient's treatment.
- They will monitor the reservoir bag to ensure that it is not being sucked in, because in this event the patient is attempting to draw more gases from the machine than is being provided. However, if it balloons, it is because the patient doesn't require the rate of gas flow being provided. In either case, the clinician must be informed and the flow rate adjusted accordingly. The second appropriate person would continue to monitor the reservoir bag in conjunction with the patient's breathing.
- If requested by the clinician, speak to the patient to reassure them. It is important to establish, before the treatment commences, who will speak to the patient while under sedation, because if both members of the team are talking at once it will compromise the patient's treatment. Potentially they will not sedate. This is because a calm, quiet atmosphere is required for inhalation sedation to be successful.

Once the patient is deemed to be satisfactorily sedated by the clinician the treatment will commence and the second appropriate person will perform the following tasks:

- Continue to monitor the patient's vital signs, demeanour and level of consciousness, paying particular attention to their respiration.
- Encourage the patient to breathe through their nose, not their mouth so that the sedation is effective.
- Constantly praise and reassure the patient throughout the period of their treatment.
- Record any changes to the percentage of nitrous oxide and oxygen administered on/in the documentation used for the patient's treatment.
- In the event that the patient experiences an emergency or they were over sedated, the second appropriate person would respond accordingly, assisting as directed by the clinician.

Once the dental treatment is complete the clinician will administer 100% oxygen for 3–5 minutes to avoid diffusion hypoxia, as explained in Chapter 5.

This must be written on/in the documentation method used to record the patient's treatment. Once complete, the mask will be removed from the patient's nose and the machine switched off. The patient can then slowly be returned to an upright position.

Role of the second appropriate person within the patient's recovery period

Patients cannot be allowed to leave the dental surgery until 20 minutes after their treatment has finished. They can either be asked to take a seat in the waiting room or the clinician may prefer them to remain in the surgery on a normal or dental chair. As soon as the patient's face has been refreshed, with all traces of treatment being removed, the second appropriate person will perform the following tasks:

- They will take all dental instruments to be sterilised and put away all materials, medicaments and equipment. They will ensure that all sharps are removed and all clinical waste is placed in the appropriate bins.
- They will continue to speak to the patient and monitor their vital signs.
- They will invite the escort, if one is present, into the dental surgery to sit with the patient and advise both the patient and escort how the treatment had progressed.
- They will take a post-operative blood pressure, if required.
- If requested by the clinician they will provide written and verbal post-operative instructions for the treatment and the sedation. This must include the telephone number of the surgery, so that if it becomes necessary, the patient or their escort can make contact.
- Once the clinician is sure that the patient is fit for discharge, the patient can leave the surgery. This is normally 20–30 minutes after completion of treatment. The second appropriate person will then record the time of discharge on/in the method of documenting the patient's treatment, write a statement of the patient's response to inhalation sedation and whether the recovery stage was uneventful. They will also record the patient's demeanour when they left the building. Once the patient has left they will carry out any unfinished cross infection control measures, tidy up and put away any items not required while preparing the dental surgery for the next patient.

ORAL SEDATION

Role of the second appropriate person when a patient is receiving treatment

As oral sedation is prescribed to be taken in a home environment, the patient must be clinically monitored and have a pulse oximeter probe placed on one

ROLE OF THE DENTAL NURSE AND EQUIPMENT

of their fingers on arrival at the surgery. This is not only because the drug provided reduces the patient's anxiety levels when attending the surgery but also because it is designed to produce sedation. Some clinicians prefer that the patient attends the surgery to take oral sedation to ensure that it has been taken correctly and that they are present should an adverse reaction occur.

Role of the second appropriate person before a patient receives treatment

The second appropriate person will perform the following tasks:

- Greet the patient and start to monitor their vital signs.
- Ask them and their escort to take a seat.
- Ask the patient the same questions and undertake the same medical checks as for intravenous sedation, because the oral sedation drugs have the same effect on the body as those administered for intravenous sedation – therefore, the patient will have the same pre-operative and post-operative restraints placed upon them.
- Record all discussions held and the outcome of the patient's medical checks on/in the documentation used to record the patient's treatment.

Role of the second appropriate person during a patient's treatment

The second appropriate person will perform the following tasks:

- They will assist with cannulation, if one is to be inserted. Placing a cannula is very good practice when using oral sedation as it will provide access into a patient's vein in the event of an emergency, over sedation or an adverse reaction. Provided patient consent has been obtained it will also allow the administration of an intravenous sedation drug if oral sedation is found to be insufficient.
- If an intravenous drug is used in conjunction with oral sedation, any amounts titrated must be documented on/in the method used to record the patient's treatment, along with the patient's percentage of saturated oxygen and pulse rate.
- They will continue to monitor the patient's vital signs, demeanour and level of consciousness, paying particular attention to their respiration, recording the percentage of saturated oxygen and pulse rate every 15–20 minutes on/in the method of documenting the patient's treatment. If any changes occur that are not within the normal limit for the patient, they will inform the clinician so that treatment can be halted and the change investigated.
- In the event that the patient experiences an emergency or they become over-sedated, the second appropriate person would respond accordingly, assisting as directed by the clinician.
- They will constantly praise and reassure the patient throughout the period of their treatment.

ROLE OF THE DENTAL NURSE AND EQUIPMENT

Role of the second appropriate person within the patient's recovery period

As soon as the patient's face has been refreshed with all traces of treatment being removed the second appropriate person will perform the following tasks:

- They will slowly raise the dental chair so that the patient is sat in the upright position.
- They will take all dental instruments to be sterilised and put away all materials, medicaments and equipment. They will ensure that all sharps are removed and all clinical waste is placed in the appropriate bins.
- If an intravenous drug was used in conjunction with oral sedation, they will dispose of any surplus, as previously explained within this chapter.
- They will record the time the treatment finished on/in the method of documenting the patient's treatment, add up and document the total amount of drug the patient received.
- On instruction from the clinician, they will invite the patient's escort into the dental surgery to sit with them and inform them how the treatment had progressed.
- They will reassure the patient, answering any questions that the patient and/or the escort may have.
- They will continue to monitor the patient's percentage of saturated oxygen and pulse rate and record on/in the method of documenting the patient's treatment.
- They will take a post-operative blood pressure if required.
- If requested by the clinician, they will provide written and verbal post-operative instructions for the treatment and sedation. This must include the telephone number of the surgery, so that if it becomes necessary, the patient or escort can make contact.
- They will assist in assessing whether the patient is fit for discharge, in the same manner as for intravenous sedation as previously explained within this chapter.
- Once the clinician is sure that the patient is fit for discharge, upon instruction/direction they will remove the cannula and place it in the sharps bin, apply pressure to the site and record the time on/in the method of documenting the patient's treatment that this occurred. The clinician may choose to remove the cannula personally – therefore, the second appropriate person will assist by providing a dressing and a sharps container.
- They will assist the patient with the help of the escort to the car.
- They will ensure that the method of documenting the patient's treatment is complete by adding the time the patient was discharged, coupled with a statement of how the patient responded while recovering.
- Once the patient has left the building the second appropriate person will carry out any unfinished cross infection control measures, tidy up and put away any items not required while preparing the dental surgery for the next patient.

TRANSMUCOSAL (OFF-LICENCE) SEDATION

Role of the second appropriate person

The second appropriate person's role and responsibilities are no different from those required for intravenous and oral sedation, as the sedation drug being used will have the same effect on the patient. The difference is that the route of administration is not the norm, or the intended route of the drug (i.e. it is placed into a drink or squirted into the patient's nose) as explained in Chapter 5.

NOTE

It is important to recognise that some clinicians prefer to undertake some of these duties themselves – therefore, the role of the second appropriate person will vary.

CLINICAL MONITORING AND EQUIPMENT USED

Monitoring a patient's vital signs is imperative when any treatment takes place to ensure that the patient is comfortable throughout and for the early detection of an emergency. The Department of Health (DH) document within its report by an expert group on sedation for dentistry states that stringent clinical monitoring must take place where all forms of sedation are administered. In the case of intravenous sedation, a pulse oximeter (Figure 3.1) and blood pressure monitor (Figure 3.27) must be used [1, 2]. The procedure of monitoring must take

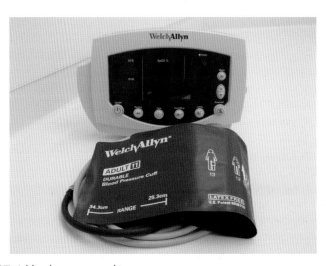

Figure 3.27 A blood pressure machine.

ROLE OF THE DENTAL NURSE AND EQUIPMENT

place as soon as the patient enters the surgery, observing the colour of their skin for comparison should the need arise and their demeanour to establish their anxiety levels. As the receptionist is the first member of the team to greet the patient they should also be capable of undertaking these simple checks. It is for this reason that they must be included in any emergency training, especially if undertaking reception duties while not being a dental nurse, so that they are able to recognise any abnormal changes while the patient is in the waiting room. By receiving this training they are able to provide first-line assistance to patients. They must alert the clinician or the dental nurse for further investigation, thereby improving the patient's chances of a speedy and full recovery. Monitoring the patient's vital signs encompasses visual checks being made as well as utilising equipment to establish the state of a patient's health.

Monitoring a patient's vital signs by observation

Although a patient's vital signs have already been documented at the assessment appointment they must be repeated on the day of their appointment. This ensures that they are still fit, healthy and able to receive treatment using a form of conscious sedation. The monitoring details are for that day only and are an aid to decide the most suitable form of sedation, according to the patient's medical fitness, expectations and required treatment. The second appropriate person must repeat these medical checks on the day of the patient's appointment so that they are in receipt of up-to-date baseline figures/recordings to work with in order that the patient can be treated and managed safely. Monitoring a patient's vital signs when sedation techniques are being used must take place throughout the appointment, with the second appropriate person observing the following:

- **Skin tone.** This must be noted as soon as the patient enters the dental surgery. The dental team is then aware of the colour, be it pale or flushed and that this is normal for that patient on the day. This avoids any unnecessary concerns (i.e. if the patient's skin colour was not noted and the team noticed it was flushed, then it might be thought that they had an allergic reaction, thus giving cause for concern). Whereas, if the dental team were aware, they would know that the skin colour had not altered. Also, if the patient was pale upon entry and this was noted, the team would not be alarmed [1].
- **The patient's demeanour.** This is noted by asking them how they are feeling that day and by observing their mannerisms. The second appropriate person must recognise whether they appear agitated or relaxed. This is important, because when a person is anxious their heart rate elevates, which places additional stress/strain on their heart. If a patient has an existing heart condition (i.e. angina), this could result in their condition occurring. A patient's blood pressure can also elevate.

- **Heart rate.** The technique employed should be manual to allow the second appropriate person to feel how strong or weak the patient's pulse is for future reference should the need arise for comparison. As explained in Chapter 7 there are many pulses within our bodies. The one to be taken is the radial pulse which is situated on the inner wrist (Figure 3.2). The second appropriate person must gently palpate that region, using the middle and index finger until they find its pulsation, count the number of beats over 30 seconds and double that figure. When feeling a pulse, the factors recorded in addition to the beats per minute are the strength and regularity, whether it is regular or irregular. If it is irregular, does it have a regular or irregular pattern? The normal pulse range for an adult is between 60 and 80 beats per minute with a resting pulse of 72. Most blood pressure machines and pulse oximeters will give a recording of the patient's pulse and it is acceptable to use these readings [1].

- **Respiratory rate.** This must be observed. It is extremely important, because the drug used for intravenous sedation has the ability to cause respiratory depression and this must be avoided. While monitoring, the second appropriate person will observe the number of breaths per minute in order to establish if the patient's breathing is within normal parameters. They will also observe the depth of respirations. They will note if the patient's breathing is shallow or if their chest expands greatly so that they are aware that this is normal for them. The procedure is quite simple. After taking the patient's heart rate by feeling the radial pulse, the second appropriate person will continue to hold the patient's wrist and then very discreetly observe the rise and fall of the chest for 30 seconds, doubling the figure obtained. The reason a patient's chest would not be looked at directly is that they would alter the depth of their respirations voluntarily, thus providing false baseline figures. A cycle of respiration is the rise and fall of the chest with a brief pause before the next cycle commences with the normal range for an adult being 12–18 breaths per minute [1].

- **Height and weight.** Some clinicians will not use conscious sedation techniques for patients above a certain body mass index. Others do not even take this figure into account. This is entirely the clinician's choice. However, it must be noted by undertaking a visual risk assessment of the patient, establishing the risk posed and associated difficulties should they have to be moved at any point while sedated. Establishing the patient's weight will prove invaluable in an emergency for calculating the amount of emergency drug to administer. Most patients are aware of their height and weight [1].

- **Temperature.** Some clinicians like to be aware of the patient's body temperature to ensure that it is normal. If elevated, treatment could be deferred, as this is indicative of an underlying fever. Normal body temperature is 37°C, which can vary slightly throughout the day. It can be taken orally over a period of 2–3 minutes ensuring that the mercury level has been shaken down, or with a digital or forehead thermometer. Patients should avoid eating, smoking or drinking for the preceding 10 minutes [1].

- **Patient's blood pressure** (Figure 3.3). This is taken to determine the patient's health/fitness to receive treatment using either an automatic machine or the manual method. Normal blood pressure is classed as approximately 120/80 or 110/70. The technique to record a patient's blood pressure is explained in detail further within this chapter [1].
- **Patient's percentage of saturated oxygen** (Figure 3.4a). This is taken using a pulse oximeter which provides readings for the second appropriate person as well as informing them of the patient's pulse rate. This is also explained in detail further within this chapter [1].
- **Patient's level of consciousness.** This is undertaken by observation and engaging the patient in conversation to ensure that they can respond, that they are not over sedated and in the case of intravenous sedation not experiencing respiratory depression. With inhalation sedation the patient should not be encouraged to talk as this can lead to ineffective sedation with gases being exhaled into the atmosphere – therefore, it will be undertaken by observation only [1].

Equipment used to monitor a patient's vital signs

While the equipment that aids monitoring is mandatory as well as valuable, it is the visual clinical monitoring that is important and the gut feeling of the team should be relied upon, not the equipment. However, that said, the second appropriate person must be able to confidently and competently use the equipment, have an understanding of their workings and be able to accurately interpret their readings [1, 2].

The equipment used include the following:

- Blood pressure machine
- Pulse oximeter

Recording a patient's blood pressure

The outcome of a patient's blood pressure is a very important diagnostic recording, as it informs the second appropriate person of the heart's activity, how well it is performing and quite simply the state of the patient's health. When blood pressure is taken prior to treatment with sedation, it is measured only once and is undertaken to establish whether it is high or low which determines the patient's fitness to receive treatment that day. Ideally, for accuracy and optimisation it should be recorded over a period of 30 minutes. The patient should not have participated in any exercise, eaten, partaken of a drink or smoked prior to this measurement and during the recording the patient should not talk. All the aforementioned can affect the outcome, as they cause the body to deal with them, thus altering the outcome and providing a false reading. Measurement should be taken in a quiet room and is achieved by using a sphygmomanometer and auscultation based on the recognition of Korotkoff sounds [1]. These are:

K1 – An audible sharp thud (systolic)
K2 – Blowing or swishing sound
K3 – Thudding sound
K4 – Muffled sound
K5 – Blood flow laminar (diastolic)

A cuff is inflated to occlude the brachial artery and as it slowly deflates the sounds can be heard with the use of a stethoscope. When recording and discussing a patient's blood pressure it is expressed as millimetres of mercury (mmHg) and is written as the systolic figure over the diastolic (i.e. 120/80). It is also referred to as systemic arterial blood pressure. There are two methods that the second appropriate person can use. One is to utilise an automatic machine and the second is to record a blood pressure manually. In order to undertake this procedure and to interpret the reading recorded the second appropriate person must have some knowledge and understanding of how a person's blood pressure is regulated [1].

What happens within the heart

The left ventricle pumps blood into the aorta. This is known as the cardiac output. The aortic walls stretch to allow increased volume. This is when the heart is at its highest pressure and provides the systolic reading. The aortic walls start to recoil, pushing blood into the arteries ensuring an onward flow. The heart at this stage is between beats. The aortic valve then closes as the pressure exceeds that of the left ventricle to prevent a backflow of blood. As the aorta and artery walls return to normal, the pressure drops to its lowest prior to the next beat which provides the diastolic reading [1].

Blood pressure

Regulation of blood pressure

It is essential that a steady flow of blood is maintained throughout the body, as it is this that will normally prevent a person fainting as they rise from a chair. Without these protective mechanisms, it would lead to an inadequate blood flow temporarily being received by the brain. The mechanisms that regulate the blood flow through the body are neural, chemical and renal. All three act together to adjust cardiac output, peripheral vascular resistance and blood volume in order to maintain an adequate blood pressure for the body's various needs. The blood pumped through the vessels is always under pressure, with this pressure at its highest within the arteries closest to the heart, gradually decreasing as the blood travels around the body. The blood keeps circulating around the body because of differences in pressure within the blood vessels and flows from high-pressure areas to low-pressure areas until it returns to the heart. Blood pressure is controlled by three things [1,3,4]:

1. Heart rate, known as the cardiac output. As a rule, when the heart rate is elevated the blood pressure will rise and when it is slower the blood pressure will drop. There are numerous factors that can affect the heart rate. These are body temperature, medication, disease, nervous system and chemical messengers, which are hormones [1,3,4].
2. Every time the heart beats blood is ejected into the aorta from the left ventricle. This is known as the stroke volume. At rest, this stroke volume equals that of the blood within the veins being returned to the heart. However, when a person is under stress the nervous system can increase the stroke volume which results in the heart pumping harder. A person's stroke volume will naturally increase or decrease the amount of blood circulating and can be altered by certain hormones, diseases and drugs [1,3,4].
3. Whether the arteries are dilated, constricted, flexible or rigid, blood entering a narrow vessel will meet more resistance than blood entering a wide vessel. When the heart pumps more blood because of the increase in stroke volume the arteries have the ability to alter their diameter, making the area wider or narrower. This prevents the blood pressure from altering drastically. This action is known as peripheral vascular resistance. Most resistance within the circulation of blood occurs within the arterioles which contain smooth muscle walls which have the ability to relax and contract, allowing the blood vessels to widen or narrow. These are important as they provide immediate regulation of blood pressure [1,3,4].

The heart

Blood pressure is determined by the force that is used to push the blood through the veins every time the heart beats and rests. If the heart pumps more blood through the arteries, or they are narrowed and stiff, the arteries will resist the blood flow. This results in blood pressure being raised and if less blood is pumped through the arteries, or they are larger and more flexible, blood pressure will be lower. The body is able to adjust the blood pressure by altering the amount of blood pumped into the arteries, the volume and viscosity of the blood and whether or not the arteries will resist that blood flow, thus regulating it. It does this by nerve impulses being sent to the heart, arteries and kidneys, so that they will, in turn, work together to make the necessary adjustments [1].

Veins and arteries

Veins and arteries can dilate to accommodate more blood when needed. This will reduce high blood pressure as the heart has less blood to pump and less is returned. They can also constrict to allow for less blood, therefore returning more blood to the heart and raising the blood pressure. The heart has to pump an increased amount of blood with more force. Similar to the heart, any adjustment to the veins and arteries will alter the blood pressure immediately [1].

The kidneys
Our kidneys have the ability to produce more or less urine to raise or lower blood pressure. More urine being produced results in less blood within the veins and arteries. Therefore the blood pressure reduces and when less urine is produced it results in more blood filling the veins and arteries, leading to an increase in blood pressure. The arteries within the kidneys determine how much salt and water is contained within the urine that passes out of the body. Enzymes produce hormones that regulate the amount of blood entering the arteries. Any increase or decrease in urine production can take weeks to make a difference to a person's blood pressure [1].

Drugs to reduce blood pressure
Drugs that reduce a person's blood pressure, for example Atenolol (beta-blocker) and Ramipril (ACE inhibitor), act upon the blood vessels to widen them, making it easier for blood to circulate without meeting resistance or cause the heart to beat less forcefully.

CONCLUSION

Any changes in a patient's cardiac output, stroke volume or peripheral vascular resistance will result in an alteration of blood pressure [1].

Technique to take a manual blood pressure

The second appropriate person will perform the following tasks:

- They will prepare a sphygmomanometer and stethoscope (Figure 3.28), ensuring that the stethoscope is switched on by turning the prongs away from their face before placing it in their ears and tapping the head.
- They will invite the patient into the room, take their coat and ensure they are seated comfortably with their arm supported (Figure 3.29).
- They will enquire if they have had their blood pressure taken before, whether they are aware of it being high or low and ask if they are taking any medication for their blood pressure.
- They will briefly explain the procedure by advising that it will take only a few minutes. They will also explain that a suitable size cuff will be placed around their upper arm and that it will initially get tight, but that the pressure will reduce quickly. The patient at this stage must be given the opportunity to ask questions.

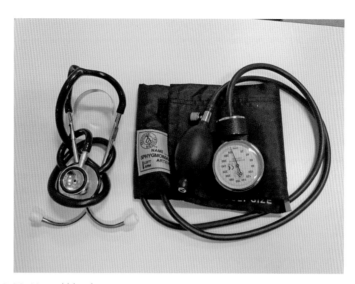

Figure 3.28 Manual blood pressure equipment.

- They will place the stethoscope around their own neck (Figure 3.30).
- They will apply the cuff to the patient's upper arm approximately 2–3cm above the antecubital fossa (Figure 3.31), ensuring that it is not too tight.
- They will take an estimated reading by palpating the radial artery (Figure 3.32), ensuring that the inflating valve is closed (Figure 3.33). They will inflate the cuff, feeling for the disappearance of the radial pulse while taking note of the sphygmomanometer level and immediately release the cuff by opening the inflating valve.

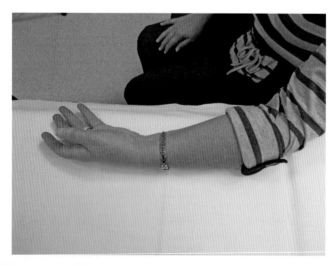

Figure 3.29 Patient's arm being supported.

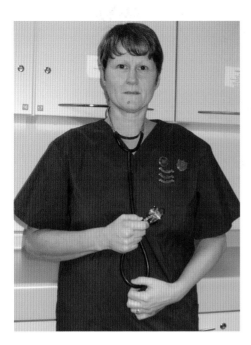

Figure 3.30 Stethoscope around nurse's neck.

- They will place the stethoscope into their own ears (Figure 3.34) and close the inflating valve.
- They will wait for 30 seconds and locate the brachial artery (Figure 3.35).
- They will place the head of the stethoscope over the brachial artery, tucking it under the cuff (Figure 3.36), applying a small amount of pressure to secure

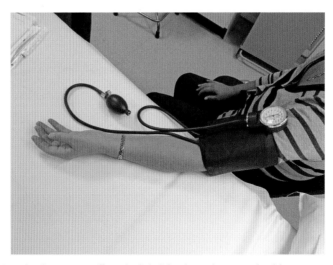

Figure 3.31 Blood pressure cuff applied slightly above the antecubital fossa.

ROLE OF THE DENTAL NURSE AND EQUIPMENT

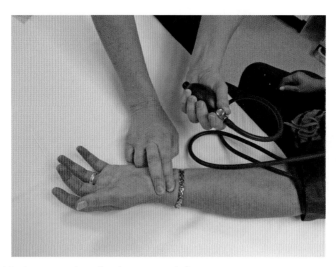

Figure 3.32 An estimated reading being recorded.

its position and holding it with their thumb over the top and their fingers on the elbow (Figure 3.37).

- They will re-inflate the cuff in order that the sphygmomanometer level rises to 30 mmHg above the estimated reading or to a maximum of 160 mmHg (Figures 3.38a and b).
- They will slowly open the inflating valve to deflate the cuff.
- They will listen for the Korotkoff sounds, taking note of the first sound and when it becomes inaudible. At this point the inflating valve must be opened to deflate the cuff.

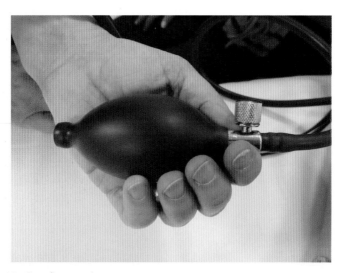

Figure 3.33 The inflating valve.

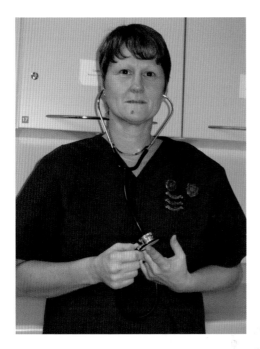

Figure 3.34 Stethoscope in nurse's ears

- They will record the outcome.
- If the blood pressure is elevated the second appropriate person would wait for 2 minutes, retake it and if still elevated ask a colleague to undertake the procedure. If all three readings are high, then the clinician would be informed so that he/she can decide whether to proceed with or defer treatment. If

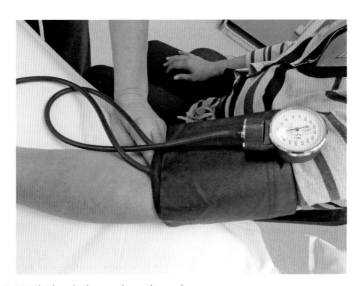

Figure 3.35 The brachial artery being located.

ROLE OF THE DENTAL NURSE
AND EQUIPMENT

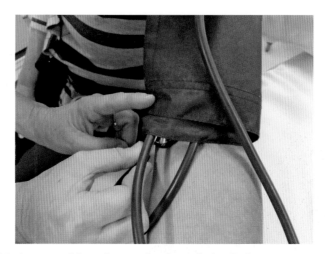

Figure 3.36 Placement of the stethoscope head over the brachial artery.

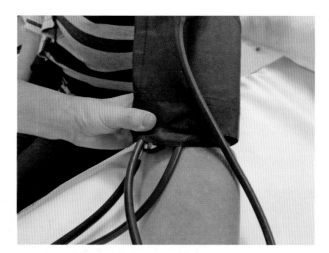

Figure 3.37 Stethoscope being held over the brachial artery.

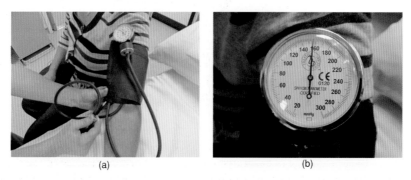

(a)   (b)

Figure 3.38 (a) Blood pressure cuff being inflated. (b) Dial at approximately 160 mmHg.

delaying treatment, the clinician may request that the patient seeks medical attention.

Technique to take an automatic blood pressure

Patient requirements and preparation are as for the manual machine.
The second appropriate person will perform the following tasks:

- Switch the machine on (Figure 3.28).
- Ensure the machine is working.
- Apply a suitable size cuff 2–3cm above the antecubital fossa.
- Press start.
- Record the reading on/in the method of documentation used for a patient's treatment.

Pulse oximetry

The use of a pulse oximeter (Figure 3.1) is mandatory when all forms of sedation take place, with the exception of inhalation sedation when it becomes the clinician's decision. It is a medical device that allows early detection of cerebral hypoxia. It indirectly measures the percentage of arterial oxygen saturation in a patient's blood, with most monitors also measuring the heart rate. The pulse oximeter displays the percentage of oxygen saturation and the pulse visually and audibly by bleeping. Many machines alter the pitch according to the oxygen saturation. A descending pitch indicates a lower saturation. This feature means that the team doesn't have to look at the display in order to establish the state of a patient's health. They can interpret a decreasing saturation by listening to the bleep. The pulse oximeter is only an aid to monitoring and should not be relied upon, as it is the clinical monitoring and judgement of the team that is paramount. It measures the 98–99% of the oxygen level within the blood that is adjoined to the haemoglobin and is measured as oxygen saturation (SaO_2). It has very little delay as it updates several times a second. It has battery backup which allows continuous monitoring in the event of power failure. It is subject to regular servicing, is portable and has a probe (Figure 3.39) which is placed over a vascular bed. The probe is normally clipped to a patient's finger (Figure 3.4a). This allows the pulse oximeter to pick up the colour of the blood as it alters from dark red to a brighter red because of the haemoglobin changing from deoxygenated to an oxygenated state. It performs this as the finger probe, also known as a photo detector, projects two lights through the finger to a receptor on the other side of the probe (Figure 3.40). This allows measurements to be taken of the intensity of each light transmitted and a comparison of the absorption of each wavelength, one against the other. The pulse oximeter then produces the percentage of saturated oxygen. This occurs because of the difference in the intensity of light absorption through the vascular bed. The difference

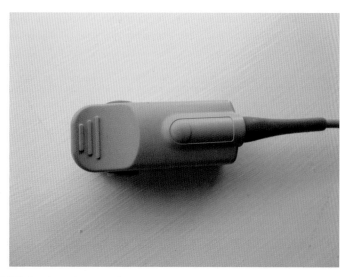

Figure 3.39 A pulse oximeter probe.

is determined by the respective levels of oxygenated and deoxygenated blood present. The optical properties change as a consequence of oxygen saturation which decreases the infrared transmission and increases the red light transmission. Pulse oximetry combines the principles of optical plethysmography and spectrophotometry. Optical plethysmography utilises technology by using light absorption to reproduce waveforms produced by the pulsatile blood known as plethysmographic waveforms. Spectrophotometry utilises scientific technology by using various wavelengths of light, performing

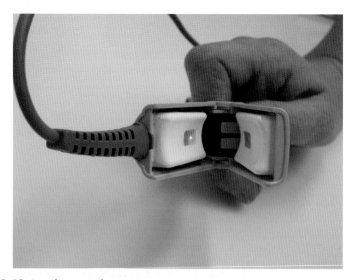

Figure 3.40 A probe opened up.

quantitative measurements of absorption through a given substance, which, in this instance, is the blood. This determines the percentage of saturation. Pulse oximeters are extremely accurate, especially within the 80–100% range of readings. Any discrepancy will only be 1–2% under the measurement. This is preferable as the patient is always more saturated than the machine indicates. This provides time, should any complications occur or if any inbuilt alarms activate. Ideally all pulse oximeters should have alarms incorporated. They can be set to activate at certain critical levels of pulse and oxygen saturation, having the facility to alter to suit the physiology of individuals. The norm is to set the low pulse level at 55 beats per minute to hopefully eradicate bradycardia (slow pulse rate), which could be indicative of an impending collapse. The high pulse level should be set at 140 beats per minute to hopefully eradicate tachycardia (fast pulse rate), which places an unnecessary strain on the heart. The low saturation level should always be set at 90. This is because levels between 90% and 100% are relatively safe as the oxygen dissociation curve (Figure 3.41) being sigmoidal shape (non-linear or S-shape) means that there is a plentiful supply of oxygen for the tissues. Below this level a rapid drop in saturation will occur. This is the result of a little change in the oxygen tension, and a state of hypoxia is reached below 85%. The oxygen dissociation curve is a graph which plots the amount of saturated haemoglobin on the vertical axis against the oxygen tension on the horizontal axis. It is a very useful resource for understanding how the blood carries and releases oxygen. The shape of the curve results from the interaction of the adjoined oxygen molecules to the haemoglobin with the incoming oxygen molecules. The haemoglobin molecule

ROLE OF THE DENTAL NURSE AND EQUIPMENT

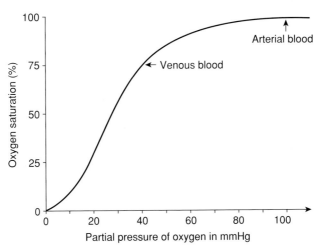

Figure 3.41 Oxygen dissociation curve. (From Ireland, R. S. (2010) *Advanced Dental Nursing*, 2nd edn. Reproduced with permission from John Wiley & Sons. (Adapted from Mallett, J. and Dougherty, L. (2000) *The Royal Marsden Hospital Manual of Clinical Nursing Procedures*, 5th edn.))

can only carry four oxygen molecules. It is very difficult for the first molecule to join, but having done so it aids the adjoining of the second and the third one. Once the fourth molecule is adjoined it is difficult to increase the level of oxygen due to overcrowding and oxygen's natural tendency to dissociate. The curve levels out as the haemoglobin becomes saturated with oxygen, giving the curve its sigmoidal or S-shape. Oxygen saturation means the volume of oxygen attached to the haemoglobin at any given time. It is related to the partial pressure of oxygen with the amount of oxygen being carried around the body. It is dependent upon the amount of haemoglobin in the blood. The curve and the theory behind it is the reason it may be difficult to achieve an increase when oxygen levels drop by encouraging the patient to take deep breaths only. Supplemental oxygen may need to be provided [1,2,5].

Clinical use

Before a patient enters the surgery the second appropriate person must ensure that the pulse oximeter is functioning properly by performing the following tasks:

- Ensure that all leads are connected properly.
- Switch the machine on to ensure that it performs a self-calibration.
- Switch off the machine to test the battery.
- Set the alarms, if in situ.
- Place it in a position that it can be seen.

Once undertaken, the probe can be placed onto a vascular bed, explaining its role to the patient. During treatment and at the recovery stage, in conjunction with visual monitoring, the second appropriate person will perform the following tasks:

- Listen to the bleep.
- Periodically observe the percentage of saturated oxygen displayed.
- If any concerns arise inform the clinician immediately.

Action to take when alarms activate and the saturation levels are below 90

Dental treatment must stop. The priority for the second appropriate person is to look at the patient to gauge if the pulse oximeter reading concurs with their clinical diagnosis. At the same time reassurance is required. The patient must be requested to take a few deep breaths. The probe must also be adjusted as it could have become dislodged. Hopefully, this is all that will be required to restore the oxygen saturation levels to a suitable percentage for the patient and treatment can resume. However, if the pulse oximeter does not concur, the patient looks well and their level of consciousness is satisfactory, another cause, whether clinical or technical, must be investigated, as explained further within this chapter. If the clinical monitoring concurs with that of the pulse oximeter the patient must be requested to take a few more deep breaths. If the patient's vital signs do not improve the airway should be checked to ensure that there is no blockage. If this doesn't rectify the situation, a head tilt, chin lift should be performed and oxygen administered. At this stage, the use of flumazenil, the emergency reversal drug, as explained in Chapter 5, will be considered by the clinician, especially if the patient's level of consciousness continues to drop. If necessary, cardiopulmonary resuscitation should be performed with the emergency services contacted. At all times the patient must be constantly monitored and reassured [1].

Clinical and technical issues

In certain conditions the pulse oximeter reading may alter. It is important for the team to recognise this, correctly interpreting the information displayed in order that they rectify the situation immediately. This hopefully avoids any complications with patient care.

Common factors that can affect the pulse oximeter measurements

Movement. A patient may tap their finger, especially if music is being played, or constantly move their hand during treatment. This can lead to changes in light absorption producing artefact pulses or changes in the saturation levels. To stop this the hand or finger could be stabilised or the probe moved to another site (i.e. ear or toe) [1].

Low perfusion. Cold hands are a common cause that can alter the pulse oximeter reading. This can lead to a false or indeed no reading being displayed, as the fingers are poorly supplied with blood when cold. Therefore, the pulse oximeter lights have a reduced amount of blood to penetrate and it is unlikely to be able to compare the ratio of the deoxygenated and oxygenated blood efficiently. To eliminate this the sensor site may be warmed prior to placement of the probe and possibly kept warm, or another site used [1].

Venous pulsation. Venous blood is not normally pulsatile, but in certain conditions of elevated venous pressure it can be (i.e. a sensor that has been too tightly applied or taped to secure it). This will result in a lower percentage of saturation or higher pulse readings. To avoid this careful positioning and securing of the sensor must take place [1].

External light source. Bright lights (i.e. the dental light shining over the sensor) can interfere with readings and can be avoided by careful movement, or the sensor could be covered with a dark drape [1].

Nail varnish. If a patient is wearing nail varnish, it should be removed as it can interfere with the readings. The machine is sensitive to blue, green, purple, black and brown nail varnish, but not red as this has, to date, never been known to interfere with the accuracy of the readings. If the patient attends wearing nail varnish, then it can be removed or the sensor placed at another site [1].

False nails. Patients should be requested not to wear false nails as they interfere with the readings. If they attend with them the probe would have to be sited elsewhere to avoid this.

Safe storage of the pulse oximeter

When treatment is complete, the pulse oximeter must be disinfected and stored safely, ensuring that it is plugged into the mains to allow battery charging.

BIBLIOGRAPHY

1. Bristol Dental Hospital course notes.
2. Department of Health, Conscious Sedation in the Provision of Dental Care, 2003.
3. www.healthmd.com/library/highbp/hbp_how.html
4. www.ehow.com/how-does-4967479_body-blood-pressure.html
5. en.wikepedia.org/wiki/Pulse_oximeter

ROLE OF THE DENTAL NURSE
AND EQUIPMENT

Chapter 4

Patient selection

LEARNING OUTCOMES

At the end of this chapter you should have a clear understanding of:

- How patients are selected for dental sedation.

INTRODUCTION

Before a patient can receive treatment with any form of conscious sedation they must attend an assessment appointment to allow the clinician to assess the patient's suitability and the method to be used for the intended treatment. Correctly managing a patient's treatment with any form of conscious sedation is essential to provide safe sedation. To do this the clinician must take into account the knowledge, skills and experience of not only himself or herself but also that of the team, as well as the express wish of the patient, coupled with their medical, dental and social history [1].

THE ASSESSMENT APPOINTMENT

It is at this appointment that the patient's treatment pathway commences, as the clinician will start to effectively manage a patient by taking and recording their medical, dental and social history. They will listen to the patient's opinions and preferences. A clinical dental examination is undertaken and any X-rays that are required are taken and assessed. The clinician will either undertake a few medical checks himself or herself or request that the dental nurse, acting as the

---

Basic Guide to Dental Sedation Nursing, First Edition. Nicola Rogers.
© 2011 Nicola Rogers. Published 2011 by Blackwell Publishing Ltd.

second appropriate person does so. The clinician may utilise a questionnaire as a tool to establish the patient's anxiety levels such as the Corah anxiety scale. The patient is asked to complete a questionnaire relating to the treatment and how they felt in certain situations before, during and after the appointment, with each question being awarded a numerical score. From the response the clinician totals the score to establish the level of the patient's concern and whether they may possibly need referral to a specialist clinician. Once in receipt of all the required information the clinician can discuss the treatment options available with the patient, take written consent and go through the pre and post-operative instructions relating to the form of sedation being provided. The patient will leave the surgery with an appointment for treatment and written pre and post-sedation instructions which he/she can refer to.

MEDICAL HISTORY

Medical history is essential in order to establish which form of sedation can safely be provided to each individual patient and whether they can be treated within a dental surgery environment or be referred to a hospital setting. When taking a medical history from a patient, a form with a list of questions covering a wide range of conditions should be given (Table 4.1). Any medical history questionnaire used should be designed to enable the patient to indicate 'yes' or 'no' to the questions to make such questionnaires user-friendly. The clinician can then discuss the information provided by the patient in more detail and if necessary, seek further clarification from the patient's doctor or a colleague who may have previously treated the patient. A clear picture of the patient's medical status can then be formed before providing treatment with any form of conscious sedation [1].

PHYSICAL EXAMINATION

Physical examination, in conjunction with medical questioning, will allow the clinician to fully assess the patient's suitability for sedation, as the outcome of this, coupled with the aforementioned, will provide enough information for the clinician to reference the American Society of Anaesthesiologists (ASA) Physical Status Classification System (Table 4.2). This enables the clinician to determine the medical risk the patient may pose while being treated with any form of conscious sedation. Only patients in ASA classes I and II should normally be dealt with in a general practice setting for treatment with sedation, with patients in ASA class III or above being referred to an appropriate secondary care establishment such as the local dental hospital. The clinician may also look

PATIENT SELECTION

Table 4.1 Medical history questions.

Central nervous system (CNS)	Epilepsy, convulsions, spastic, subnormal psychiatric problems, migraine Drug, alcohol dependency, other neurological disease
Cardiovascular system (CVS)	Heart disease, hypertension, syncope, rheumatic fever, chorea, brucellosis, bleeding disorder, anticoagulants, anaemia
Respiratory system (RS)	Asthma, bronchitis, TB, smoking, other chest diseases
Gastrointestinal (GI)	Gastric or duodenal ulcer, bleeding PR, other GI disease, hepatitis, jaundice
Gastrourinary (GU)	Renal, urinary tract or sexually transmitted disease, menstrual problems, pregnancy
Locomotor (LM)	Bone or joint disease, diabetes or other endocrine disease, skin disease or any other disease, including congenital abnormality, family relevant medical history, allergies (i.e. penicillin), recent or current drugs/medical treatment, previous operations or serious illnesses, recent travel abroad

at extending the appointment to allow for potential complications, taking into account the medical history and/or carrying out less treatment in one session so that it is less stressful for the patient [1, 2].

The examinations that should take place are explained in detail in Chapter 3 and comprise the following:

- Blood pressure (BP)
- Heart rate
- Respiratory rate
- Temperature
- Height
- Weight
- Oxygen saturation

DENTAL HISTORY

The clinician will establish the patient's past and present dental history by inviting them to discuss previous experiences and any relevant details of their current dental problem. These factors are important, as they could be detrimental to effective management. Patient's expectations must also be taken into account as they may not be realistic, especially if they request that they want to be asleep throughout the period of treatment, as conscious sedation will not provide this. A clinical examination, with or without radiographs, will give a picture of the patient's dental health and their motivation in maintaining

PATIENT SELECTION

Table 4.2 The American Society of Anaesthesiologists (ASA) Physical Status Classification System.

Classification	Patient group	Examples
ASA I	Patients who are normal and healthy Able to walk up a flight of stairs easily Physiologically should present no difficulty in handling the proposed treatment A candidate for any sedation technique	
ASA II	Patients with mild systemic disease Healthy, but present with extreme fear/anxiety towards dentistry Older, (i.e. 60 years and above) Pregnant Have to rest after mild exercise Less stress tolerant, but still represent a minimal risk during treatment Proceed with caution	Healthy patients, 60 years plus Healthy, but very phobic Non-insulin controlled diabetic Mildly raised BP, (i.e. 140–159/90–94 mmHg) History of atopic allergies
ASA III	Patients with systemic disease that limits activity, but is not incapacitating Not stressed at rest, but have to stop frequently during mild exercise, (i.e. walking or climbing stairs) Sedation procedure may need modifying/shortening or kept lighter	Well controlled insulin controlled diabetic Myocardial infarction 6 months previously with no symptoms since High BP, (i.e. 160–190/95–114 mmHg) Fragile asthmatic Epileptic with several seizures a year
ASA IV	Patients who have an incapacitating disease that is threatening to life Unable to walk upstairs or far along the street Exhibit fatigue or shortness of breath while seated Treatment should be avoided or carried out as conservatively as possible, or referred to a suitable hospital department	Unstable angina Recent myocardial infarction Poorly controlled diabetic Very high BP, (i.e. 200/115 mmHg)
ASA V	Patients with a terminal condition and not expected to survive Not suitable for treatment	
ASA VI	A declared brain dead patient whose organs are being removed for donor purposes	

good oral health. It must be remembered that complex treatments may require future maintenance. With this in mind the patient's attendance pattern must be looked at when providing treatment of this nature and it must be recognised that they may, if requiring further treatment, request additional sedation for it to be undertaken [1].

SOCIAL HISTORY

Social history is as important as the other histories taken, because the clinician has a duty of care to ensure that the patient will be adequately cared for at home. The clinician should instruct the patient to be accompanied by a responsible adult who will act as their escort on the day of their appointment, stay with them and look after them for the following 24 hours. If this is not possible then another mode of sedation would be offered. They will be advised that if they arrive without an escort then treatment will not take place. Travel arrangements will be discussed so that the patient can arrange for someone to drive them on the day of their appointment. If this is not possible, the patient should be advised to book a taxi and not to use public transport. The clinician will also decide if the patient is competent to consent to treatment, and if not, source other means of securing consent, which are explained in Chapter 2. Cost is another factor that has to be considered. It is to be ascertained whether the patient can afford to proceed or not, and if not, other ways of managing their dental care have to be explored [1].

CONCLUSION

All three histories must be documented and considered so that the patient receives the most suitable form of sedation for the intended treatment. If any one of the histories is not undertaken then patient care would be compromised. The form of conscious sedation provided must reflect the patient's needs, their wishes and personal circumstances (i.e. a patient requests intravenous sedation but has small children and no family support). As they would not have any home support/care this form of sedation would not be provided, but inhalation sedation would be offered as an alternative as it does not attract the same rigid instructions.

PATIENT SELECTION

BIBLIOGRAPHY

1. Bristol Dental Hospital course notes.
2. en.wikipedia.org/wiki/American_Society_of_Anesthesiologist

Chapter 5
Types of sedation

LEARNING OUTCOMES

At the end of this chapter you will have a clear understanding of:

- The various modes of sedation provided to patients.
- The way each mode is administered and acts upon the body.
- The advantages, disadvantages, indications and contraindications of usage.

INTRODUCTION

Patients are offered different modes of sedation depending upon their medical, dental and social history, preference, cost and team experience. The mode chosen is identified through an assessment appointment and all modes are independent of each other but can be used in conjunction. All modes of sedation act on the body differently, with the patient having to comply with the different restraints of each mode to enable them to receive it. The common forms of dental sedation provided to patients are:

- Intravenous
- Off-licence (transmucosal) sedation (It is an advanced technique which should only be used in exceptional circumstances.)
- Inhalation
- Oral sedation (It is not widely used but plays an important role within the provision of treatment with or without other forms of sedation as it reduces anxiety [1].)

Basic Guide to Dental Sedation Nursing, First Edition. Nicola Rogers.
© 2011 Nicola Rogers. Published 2011 by Blackwell Publishing Ltd.

INTRAVENOUS SEDATION

A cannula is placed into a vein and a drug is administered directly into the patient's blood stream which results in sedation. The drug used is titrated (given) according to the patient's response and is age related, not weight related as is a general anaesthetic. The most widely used drug is midazolam (Hypnovel). It belongs to the family of benzodiazepines drugs and its clinical actions and advantages are:

- It is anxiolytic to reduce a patient's anxiety levels.
- It is hypnotic to induce sleep.
- It is anticonvulsant to reduce the risk of a convulsive fit.
- It is a muscle relaxant.
- It produces anterograde amnesia. The patient will be aware of treatment but may not remember anything after the first increment of drug.
- It lowers the blood pressure and in return the body responds by raising the pulse rate to increase the cardiac output, thus raising the blood pressure.
- Less pain is experienced at the injection site.
- It results in sedation, thus allowing treatment to take place.
- It causes slurred speech and impaired coordination, indicating that the patient is sedated enough to commence treatment.
- It has a rapid onset with a pronounced effect and is short acting.
- It is water soluble, so a non-irritant.
- It can be titrated to produce a desired effect to reflect individual patient's needs.
- As a patient's vein is continually maintained drugs can be provided in the event of an emergency or if the patient becomes over sedated.
- Patient recovery time is faster than with oral or intramuscular drugs.
- Nausea and vomiting rarely occur.
- It reduces the gag reflex slightly [1, 2].

    Its disadvantages are:

- Venepuncture is mandatory and therefore needle phobics are not always conducive or cooperative to this form of sedation.
- Training is required to undertake venepuncture and it requires great skill.
- The site of venepuncture can cause problems.
- An experienced second appropriate person must be available to clinically monitor the patient at all times.
- It can cause respiratory depression to reduce the respiratory drive.
- It can have a minimal effect on the cardiovascular system (depressing it).
- Due to the rapid onset of midazolam, its action and its more pronounced effects, the risk of any potential complication is elevated.
- It does not provide any analgesia, therefore a local anaesthetic would be required for pain relief where applicable.

TYPES OF SEDATION

- Paradoxical effects occasionally occur in children and the elderly.
- Appointment times need to be longer to allow for the patient's recovery period.
- Consent must be taken, with every eventuality being considered, discussed and agreed prior to its provision.
- Patients must be able to comply with the rigid pre and post-operative instructions that intravenous sedation attracts. Most clinicians will give very similar instructions to patients. However, some may give additional instructions or alternatives that are their preference and/or specific to their area of work. Generic instructions are:
  - To be accompanied by a responsible adult to act as an escort. This person must remain at the surgery while treatment takes place and accompany the patient home by car. They must also be able to stay with the patient for the next 24 hours and be free of other responsibilities. The reason: The clinician has a duty of care to ensure that when a patient leaves the surgery they are adequately supervised and cared for so that they come to no harm.
  - Not to be in charge of other people on the day of sedation. The reason: To allow the patient to rest and recover from treatment.
  - Not to make any responsible decisions or sign any legal documents for the remainder of the day. The reason: It may not be remembered.
  - Not to drive any vehicle, operate machinery, climb ladders or scaffolding. The reason: It is illegal to drive under the influence of drugs – judgement and coordination will be impaired.
  - Not to eat or drink for 4 hours prior to the appointment time. Some clinicians do not request their patients to be starved of food and drink but advise a light meal a few hours prior to the appointment. The reason: When a person is starved of food and drink they are more difficult to cannulate as they could be dehydrated, plus they could collapse due to lack of food.
  - To wear loose clothing with sleeves that can easily be pulled above the elbow and not to wear high-heel shoes. The reason: Tight clothing restricts breathing making it more difficult to monitor and once sedation is complete it is preferable for the patient to be wearing flat shoes to avoid the risk of stumbling.
  - To remove any nail varnish. The reason: It can interfere with the pulse oximeter, giving an incorrect reading.
  - To avoid alcohol on the day of sedation. The reason: Alcohol will potentiate (speed up) the sedation drug.
  - To ensure that their teeth and gums are clean. A clean mouth heals more quickly [1, 2].

Midazolam (Hypnovel)

Midazolam is a short-acting benzodiazepine, one of approximately 35 benzodiazepines which are currently being used medically as sedative drugs. Although

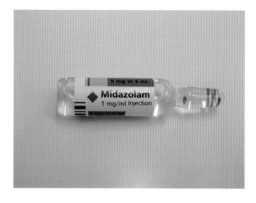

Figure 5.1 Ampoule of midazolam.

it was produced in the 1970s, it didn't become available for use until the 1980s. In the 1990s it was accepted that it was very effective in the management of status epilepticus and could be administered intramuscularly. It is a clear odourless liquid in glass ampoules that can be obtained as:

- 10mg in 5ml
- 10mg in 2ml
- 5mg in 5ml (Figure 5.1)

The recommended presentation for use in the dental surgery is 5mg in 5ml as this helps to prevent the risk of over sedation. Each box obtained will contain glass ampoules of midazolam that are stamped with the name, concentration, expiry date and the batch number (Figure 5.2). Midazolam is a controlled drug, and should, be under lock and key and treated as such with the ampoules being stored in the outer carton to protect them from light [1, 2].

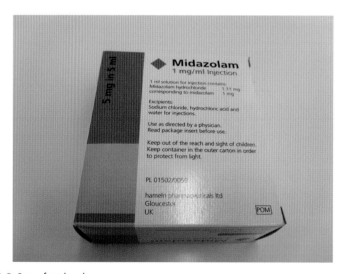

Figure 5.2 Box of midazolam.

TYPES OF SEDATION

Pharmacology (action within the body)

Within the central nervous system (CNS) there are benzodiazepine receptors that allow benzodiazepine drugs to bind to them. These receptors are parallel to gamma-aminobutyric acid (GABA) receptors. Benzodiazepine does not directly activate GABA receptors but enhances the effect of neurotransmitters on the GABA receptors resulting in inhibition of brain activity. Therefore, conscious sedation is achieved by midazolam acting on the CNS thus reducing the excitability of the neurons in the mid brain, resulting in either the slowing down or stopping of certain nerve signals with the brain. All drugs have a half-life. This means the time it takes for the plasma level of the drug to drop to half. Benzodiazepines have two stages which form their half-life and comprise the following:

- **Alpha: Distribution and redistribution.** This is where the drug is introduced into the body, taken to the brain and then redistributed to other areas of the body.
- **Beta: Metabolism and excretion.** This is where the drug is broken down by the body and eliminated.

The distribution (alpha) half-life of midazolam is 4–18 minutes with the elimination (beta) half-life being 1–4 hours. Approximately 5mg of drug will be eliminated from the body within 5 hours. However, in the elderly and adolescents the elimination half-life is longer. When midazolam is titrated, it is thought to go through four phases of sedation very quickly with the patient reaching phase IV after an hour [1–3].

Phases of sedation

Phase I

The midazolam within the blood at the site of the brain is at its maximum – therefore it is at this point that the sedation technique will also be at its maximum. This will result in the patient's coordination being impaired and their speech slurred. These signs of sedation can be established by talking to the patient, noting the change in their speech and requesting that they touch their nose. If they are successful in touching their nose they are classed as Eve sign negative and therefore not sedated sufficiently, but if they are unable to locate their nose they are Eve sign positive and sedated enough to commence treatment. At this stage the patient will be unaware of their surroundings and the team and will experience/notice a period of almost total amnesia, despite them conversing quite normally [1, 2].

Phase II

As the amount of midazolam within the blood will now start to decrease so will the effects of sedation. This is attributed to the midazolam being redistributed to other tissues within the body (alpha half-life). As a result, the patient will experience an awareness of their surroundings and the team as the amnesic effect decreases. This means that some patients may remember parts of their treatment [1,2].

Phase III

It is at this stage that the patient will start to feel normal and will still appear to look relaxed. They will not be anxious as the anxiolytic effect of midazolam is still active. They will not experience any pain because of the numbing effects of the local anaesthetic [1,2].

Phase IV

The patient will look and feel recovered. It must be remembered that the patient is not fully recovered at this stage as it is only the alpha half-life (distribution and redistribution) that has occurred. The midazolam has yet to undergo the beta half-life (metabolism and excretion) and is therefore still present within the body. The amnesic effects of midazolam must also not be forgotten. They can be profound enough to last until phase IV of the sedation, meaning that the post-operative instructions must be reiterated and always provided in writing to both the patient and escort [1,2].

Administration of midazolam

If a patient has received previous treatment with intravenous sedation, well-written notes will provide an indication of how well the patient responded and the amount they received. The dose titrated can then be adjusted accordingly. The usual administration of midazolam for a young person who is classified as an ASA I (as explained in Chapter 4) is:

- Initial bolus of 2mg over 30 seconds. Patient response will be observed and monitored for 2 minutes.
- After 2 minutes, a further 0.5–1mg is administered until the level of sedation required has been achieved, with the usual dose being between 2.5 and 7.5mg.

As the elderly are much more sensitive to midazolam its administration must be slower, allowing longer periods between the titrations. This avoids over sedation with the initial bolus being slowly administered over 2 minutes with the dose being as low as 1–1.5mg. The total amount of midazolam given may not need to exceed 3.5mg. The reason is that elderly patients' arm brain time is much slower than that of younger patients. If midazolam is titrated in the same way to an elderly patient it could lead to over sedation. Upon administration of midazolam the elderly patient may not appear sedated as it takes longer for the dose to travel to the brain than that of the younger patient. If further increments of midazolam are administered the initial dose will eventually reach the brain. This initial dose may have been enough to sedate the patient. However, the body still contains the additional increments and they will not have yet reached the brain. Once they do, it could result in an over sedated patient [1].

Side effects of midazolam

All drugs can cause side effects with many patients experiencing minor symptoms to intravenous midazolam. These are:

- Minimal cardiovascular effects
- Respiratory effects
- Hiccoughs
- Coughing
- Headaches
- Drowsiness
- Nausea and vomiting
- Loss of inhibition
- Restlessness
- Irritation at the cannula site (However, as midazolam is water soluble it is not common for the patient to experience any irritation [1,2].)

Special precautions and some contraindications of usage
Pregnancy and the nursing mother

As with all drugs, using midazolam on a pregnant patient is not recommended as it is known to slowly cross the placental barrier to enter the fetal blood. If used, it would be likely that the effects would manifest in the fetus and if used regularly in the third trimester it could lead to the baby experiencing benzodiazepine withdrawal syndrome. If a nursing mother is breastfeeding and receives treatment with intravenous sedation she would have to express enough breast milk prior to the treatment to last for 24 hours and to avoid breast feeding for the same period. If she does not undertake this the baby would receive traces of midazolam from her milk when feeding [1–3].

Kidney or liver impairment

This could slow down the rate at which midazolam is eliminated from the body resulting in prolonged and enhanced effects [1–3].

The elderly

As previously explained, elderly patients are more sensitive to the effects of midazolam. They may also metabolise and eliminate it much slower and are potentially more at risk to prolonged drowsiness, amnesia, hangover effects, confusion and accidental falls [1–3].

Children

The use of intravenous midazolam for children is not recommended as they may exhibit a paradoxical effect (i.e. agitation, involuntary movement and hyperactivity) [1].

Allergy to benzodiazepines

If a patient has a hypersensitivity to benzodiazepines, or any constituents thereof, it should not be used. In the event that this is unknown and a patient experiences a reaction, then the administration of the drug should be stopped, the patient's airway maintained, oxygen provided and adrenaline administered. As the patient will have an indwelling cannula the intravenous concentration of adrenaline can be provided, which is 0.5ml 1:10,000. Flumazenil must never be given as it would increase the anaphylactic reaction.

Alcohol and drug abuse

Benzodiazepines should be used with extreme caution in patients who have a history of alcohol abuse as the effects of the alcohol can potentiate (speed up) the effect of the drug. There is also a risk that the patient may have liver impairment which could prolong the elimination of the midazolam. Patients with a history of drug abuse may be difficult to cannulate and thus other sites may have to be used. They may also be more difficult to sedate, requiring larger doses. As with any substance that depresses the central nervous system and/or provides any muscle-relaxant effects particular care should be taken when administering midazolam (i.e. in the case of myasthenia gravis, as these patients have pre-existing muscle weakness) [2,3].

Cardiorespiratory disorders

Effects associated with cardiovascular disorders are rare but can occur and include effects such as respiratory depression, apnoea, respiratory arrest and/or cardiac arrest. These life threatening incidents are more likely to occur in patients over 60 years of age and with those who have pre-existing respiratory insufficiency or impaired cardiac function, particularly when the injection is given too rapidly or when a high dose of midazolam is administered [1].

Analgesics and midazolam

Opiates, normally Nubain (nalbuphine), can be, but are very rarely used in conjunction with midazolam to enhance sedation effects. The use of two intra-venous drugs being titrated together is known as polypharmacy. The reason it may be used is for the provision of additional post-operative pain relief for patients. However, the use of a long-acting local anaesthetic is usually sufficient and eliminates the need for their use. Nubain should be administered first as it

TYPES OF SEDATION

is not titrated but given in one dose. This means that midazolam can be safely titrated on top of any sedation induced by the analgesic. Patients who receive both drugs tend to experience sleepiness, nausea and vomiting and can experience profound respiratory depression. If an emergency occured, Nubain's reversal drug Narcan (naloxone) would be administered [3].

Erythromycin

It inhibits the metabolism of midazolam resulting in a prolonged effect [2].

St John's wort

It enhances the metabolism of midazolam resulting in a reduced effect [2].

Potential complications

- The wrong drug administered, due to failure to check the ampoule contents, lack of drug labelling or incorrect labelling.
- Drug out of date due to the expiry date not being checked or recorded on the patient's treatment pathway documentation.
- Allergic reaction due to patient sensitivity to the drug not being known or recorded in the patient's notes.
- Venepuncture complication (i.e. extravasation where the cannula has been inserted into the vein and exits the other wall, meaning that when the drug is titrated a swelling like a fried egg will occur in that area). To treat this, administration of the drug should be stopped and depending upon the clinician the cannula will be either left or removed and if removed, pressure will be applied to the area. Bruising can occur on insertion or removal of a cannula. This is usually attributed to poor venepuncture technique upon insertion and lack of pressure being applied upon removal. Collapse of the vein during cannulation. This is difficult to overcome and is normally attributed to patient anxiety. To avoid these and other complications the right anatomical site should be chosen along with the correct size cannula and the tourniquet should be secured tightly with the chosen limb adequately restrained. It is very important that the patient is monitored and reassured and the clinician will of course be decisive regarding the success or failure of the cannula's placement. Upon removal, pressure applied to the cannulation site must be undertaken by the clinician or second appropriate person and not the patient.
- The cannula comes out due to it not being secured properly, meaning that the continual access required to administer further increments of midazolam and more importantly for the administration of a drug or drugs should an emergency occur has been lost.
- Inadequate post-sedation supervision. The patient was not fit for discharge when they left the dental surgery or the escort either did not attend or was unsuitable. If an escort is not in attendance, treatment should be postponed.

- Over sedation, which is recognised by the patient's chin dropping and lack of response to verbal commands [1].

Overdose of midazolam

The signs and symptoms that a patient would exhibit if they were over sedated are: Drowsiness, mental confusion, lethargy and muscle relaxation. They would not respond if they were asked a question or would not rouse if tapped on the shoulder. An overdose of midazolam should not be life threatening unless it has been combined with other central nervous system depressants, which includes alcohol. More serious signs and symptoms would be hypotension, cardiorespiratory depression, apnoea and rarely, a coma. Careful titration of midazolam, coupled with good patient management and comprehensive clinical monitoring, can prevent over sedation.

Treatment of an overdose of midazolam

Careful observation of the patient's vital signs is required, coupled with airway maintenance and the provision of oxygen. The benzodiazepine antagonist flumazenil (Anexate) will be used to control the effects of over sedation. This emergency drug must always be available when intravenous sedation takes place with the minimum of two vials being held. The maximum dose a patient can receive is 1mg. If necessary cardiopulmonary resuscitation will be undertaken and the emergency services called [1].

Flumazenil (Anexate)

This is a clear liquid, obtained as 500 micrograms (mcg) in a 5ml glass ampoule with the name, batch number, expiry date and quantity of drug stamped on each ampoule (Figures 5.3 and 5.4). It is the antidote for an overdose of a benzodiazepine and is an imidazobenzodiazepine derivative, which antagonises the clinical actions of benzodiazepines on the central nervous system. The pharmacology of flumazenil is that it competitively inhibits the activity at the

TYPES OF SEDATION

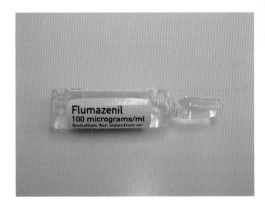

Figure 5.3 Ampoule of flumazenil.

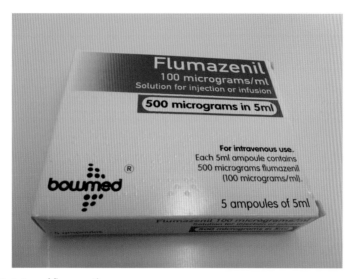

Figure 5.4 Box of flumazenil.

benzodiazepine GABA receptors. This allows the neurons to return to their normal state of excitability, thus reversing the sedative effect. Flumazenil is a controlled drug, be kept under lock and key and treated as such with the ampoules being stored in the outer carton to protect them from light [1,6].

Administration of flumazenil

It is titrated as follows:

- 200mcg over 15 seconds.
- If required, further doses of 100mcg are repeated every minute until the desired level of consciousness has been achieved.

The maximum dose is 1mg, which is two vials. The usual dose administered is 300–600mcg [1].

Effects of flumazenil

The patient may exhibit and experience the following effects:

- Anxiety
- Disorientation
- Head pains
- Aggressiveness
- Agitation [1]

Re-sedation

Patients who have received flumazenil for the reversal of benzodiazepine effects should be monitored for re-sedation and respiratory depression for an appropriate period. This is because the half-life of flumazenil is approximately 50 minutes and the half-life of midazolam is 1–4 hours. Therefore, it is conceivable that when used to reverse the action of midazolam the patient will initially be reversed, but could become re-sedated as the action of flumazenil decreases. However, very little re-sedation will occur as both drugs will wear off together. Once broken down flumazenil is excreted in urine. Any patient who has received flumazenil to reverse the effects of midazolam must be warned that the post-operative care instructions are still applicable. They must also be kept in the surgery for a suitable period of time and be assessed for discharge before being allowed to leave the surgery [1,6].

Some contraindications of usage
Patients dependent on benzodiazepines

If patients who rely on benzodiazepine medication for medical conditions become over sedated when reversing the effects of midazolam the effects of their medication will be reversed as well.

Coronary heart disease

When treating patients who have heart conditions with midazolam their anxiety levels are reduced, thus reducing the strain placed on their heart when they are in stressful situations. If the effects of the sedation are reversed they will be placed very quickly into the situation/environment that was being avoided by sedating them. They would be very anxious and their heart rate would increase, placing unnecessary strain on it.

Epileptic patients

Patients who suffer from epilepsy are prescribed medication that belongs to the benzodiazepine family. Therefore, when the action of the midazolam is reversed so will their epileptic therapy, resulting in the patient experiencing convulsions [1].

Propofol (Diprivan)

Propofol is widely used in hospital settings. It is not commonly used for dental sedation in a general practice, as it is used by anaesthetists to induce and maintain patients receiving a general anaesthetic. The recovery time with its use is rapid. It provides patients with amnesic and hypnotic effects and reduces the chance of a patient vomiting. It works by enhancing the effect of GABA to depress the central nervous system without using the receptors directly. It is

TYPES OF SEDATION

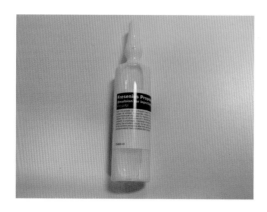

Figure 5.5 Ampoule of propofol.

a white, milky liquid which is obtained in glass ampoules of 200mg in 20ml (10mg per ml) (Figure 5.5). It has a rapid onset and quick recovery with the half-life being estimated between 2 and 24 minutes and patient recovery being within 5 minutes. For dental sedation propofol is used with a patient controlled electronic infusion pump driver so that it can be continually administered (Figure 5.6). These drivers are similar to those used after general surgery for post-operative pain relief in general hospitals. The pump driver is set up by the clinician or the anaesthetist by inputting the amount of drug a patient will receive each time they press a button and the interval period between activations. This means that the patient is in control, because they hold the button throughout treatment, which when pressed will administer a dose of propofol. Due to the data input (hence the lockout time), they would not

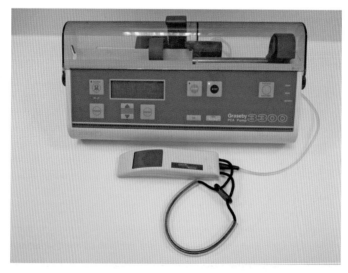

Figure 5.6 Pump driver.

receive a dose every time they press the button. Injection of propofol can be painful – therefore, it should be administered into larger veins or following a pre-injection with a local anaesthetic. As the margin between sedation and anaesthesia is far narrower than that of midazolam, it must be remembered that when administering any general anaesthetic agent it has to be undertaken where appropriately trained staff and facilities for monitoring patients are available. Proper airway management, together with a supply of supplemental oxygen, artificial ventilation and cardiovascular resuscitation must also be available. Propofol attracts the same pre and post-operative instructions as midazolam and is a controlled drug, should be under lock and key and treated as such with the ampoules being stored in the outer carton to protect them from light [1,9].

Some contraindications of usage
Patient prescribed respiratory depressants

Propofol is potentiated by these drugs [9].

Pregnancy and the nursing mother

As with all drugs, using propofol for a pregnant patient is not recommended, as it is known to slowly cross the placental barrier to enter the fetal blood.

Patients who are allergic to eggs

Propofol is an emulsion which is dissolved in a soya-bean oil, glyceryl and purified egg – therefore, these patients would suffer an anaphylactic reaction [9].

Transmucosal (off-licence) sedation

The off-licence use of a drug means that it is being used in an alternative way to that for which it has been researched, tried and tested. This form of sedation is classed as an advanced technique, as the clinician has no control over the absorption of the drug within the body. If midazolam was being used by a clinician in this way and an adverse reaction or incident occurred, he/she could be open to question/investigation to establish why this technique was adopted. If used it should only be administered in appropriate circumstances and setting. This mode of sedation is very useful in the management of special needs patients and needle phobics. The routes used for transmucosal midazolam are:

- Oral
- Nasal

Due to midazolam's bitter taste when administered orally it needs to be added to either cold tea, apple juice or a sweetened fruit juice to mask its taste. If used in this way a patient would be given the drink at their appointment with

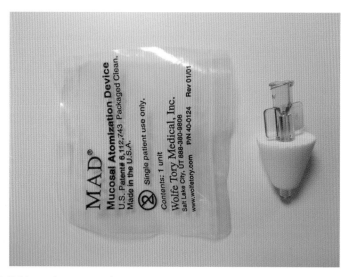

Figure 5.7 Mucosal atomising device.

its sedative effect occurring within approximately 20 minutes. When providing patients with intranasal midazolam, a mucosal atomising device (Figure 5.7) is used to place the midazolam, as when squirted it provides a fine aerosol allowing the drug to be directed up the nose for absorption. It is thought that the onset of the sedative effect through the nasal route is slightly faster than that through the oral route. The same intravenous pre and post-operative restrictions will apply to patients, as does the level of care provided by the team. Some clinicians using off-licence sedation place a cannula, so that if required, they can administer further increments of midazolam and very importantly would have one in situ should an emergency arise. If a cannula is not placed and it becomes necessary, then the clinician would place and secure one immediately. However, buccal midazolam is available and licensed for the management of status epilepticus. It is a sugar-free liquid called Epistatus available as 10mg per 1ml. It is placed against the sides of the gingiva and cheek, being absorbed directly into the bloodstream. There is no need for it to be swallowed, but if it is, it may not be as effective. This method offers the opportunity for clinicians to use it for sedation or as a pre-medication to allow cannulation to take place [7, 8].

INHALATION SEDATION

Also known as relative analgesia. This form of sedation is considered to be the least invasive that can be administered to patients receiving treatment, as there

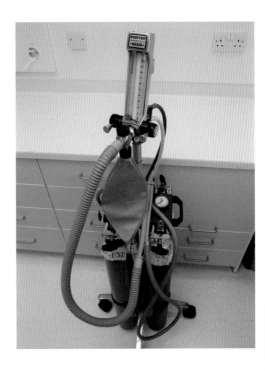

Figure 5.8 Mobile relative analgesia machine.

is no need to place a cannula. This is because patients are sedated via their respiratory system so there are no post-operative restraints for the patient to comply with. It is widely used to provide treatment to children as these factors make it an ideal mode of sedation. A relative analgesia machine is required to administer an appropriate amount of nitrous oxide, together with oxygen to produce a sedated/euphoric state. Machines used can be either mobile or piped systems (Figures 5.8 and 5.9). When used to sedate patients for treatment it must be in a quiet environment with the clinician using sympathetic hypnotic suggestion for it to be successful. It is important that the team know their patient so that if they reference something to relax them the patient does not associate it with any bad experiences. An acclimatisation visit is very useful to prepare the patient for their treatment session, as this allows them to become familiar with the equipment. The patient will try on various masks in order to establish the correct size. If the patient is happy the chosen mask can be used to supply a short exposure of oxygen. In this way they are made aware of the nasal sensations they will experience. The fact that it is non-invasive and relatively safe does not negate the need for staff to be well trained with the same requirements being in place as for intravenous sedation in respect of patient care. When providing patients with inhalation sedation it improves patient cooperation, as their levels of anxiety are reduced, allowing treatment to take place [1].

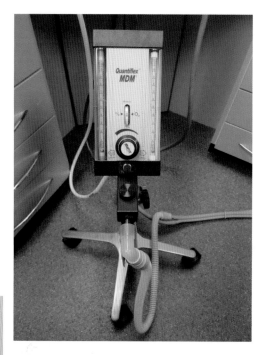

Figure 5.9 Piped relative analgesia machine.

Advantages of inhalation sedation

The advantages of inhalation sedation are:

- Its use is extremely safe as it is a non-invasive technique, because an indwelling cannula is not required to inject a drug. There is no gastric absorption or any significant metabolism – therefore there would be no adverse effects on the liver, kidneys, brain, cardiovascular or respiratory system. There is minimal impairment of the cough and swallowing reflexes so the patient's airway is not compromised. Patients recover very quickly and there are no post-sedation restrictions so they can undertake any of their normal responsibilities/activities. One of the key factors that make it a safe form of sedation is that at all times a patient receives a minimum of 30% oxygen. This is 10% more than in atmospheric air – therefore a patient cannot receive any more than 70% nitrous oxide.
- The patient will feel its effect within 20 seconds and within 3–5 minutes will experience its full effect.
- The length of the patient's appointment can reflect the treatment being undertaken. It is ideal for long or short procedures and it can be provided for all ages with very few contraindications.
- It can be accurately delivered to patients with the amount of nitrous oxide and oxygen being altered to suit their needs. When altering the depth of sedation, it takes approximately 2–3 minutes for a change to be noticed.

TYPES OF SEDATION

- The nitrous oxide sedates while providing some analgesia and anterograde amnesia with the latter not as profound as intravenous sedation [1].

Disadvantages of inhalation sedation

The disadvantages of inhalation sedation are:

- The team must provide psychological support to patients to achieve successful sedation. Its use and success are reliant on a patient-centred approach, good communication and the power of gentle coercion. Coupled with reasoning, trust is then engendered. This can be difficult with some categories of patients such as the medically compromised. However, that said, the depth of sedation can vary between patients and can even differ for the same patient at other appointments. It is therefore important for the team to know their patient and which supportive techniques work for individuals.
- If a patient has a cold or cannot breathe properly through his/her nose on the day they must cancel their appointment. This is because the sedation will be ineffective as its action is through the respiratory system. Also the gases used are under positive pressure. They could push the patient's upper respiratory tract infection further into their respiratory system.
- Nitrous oxide is not very potent – therefore some patients will not achieve a suitable level of sedation for treatment to take place.
- The cost of providing this form of sedation is high as the equipment is expensive and requires ongoing servicing and maintenance, plus the continuous use of the gases.
- Whether a mobile machine or a piped system is used they are awkward in shape. This makes space and storage an issue. If a mobile machine is used the cylinders have to be stored securely so additional safe storage is required.
- Long-term exposure to nitrous oxide can cause harm to the team – therefore control measures must be put in place, coupled with the use of a scavenging system to remove it, thereby limiting the risk of a harmful effect. It cannot be used without oxygen, with a minimum of 30% provided by the machine at all times to avoid the risk of death. Unfortunately, it is very accessible to the team so there is a risk of recreational abuse [1].

TYPES OF SEDATION

Pharmacology (action within the body)

A patient receives nitrous oxide and oxygen through a nasal mask by inhaling these gases into the respiratory system until they reach the alveoli sacs within the lungs. This is where the gaseous exchange takes place. One of the characteristics of both gases is that they will always down the gradient. They will always move towards an area that doesn't contain as much of the same gas, thus working comparable to breathing when eliminating carbon dioxide from the body and taking oxygen. When we breathe the blood within the lungs has no oxygen and it contains high levels of carbon dioxide with the atmospheric air within the lungs being the reverse. Based on the aforementioned characteristic of gases the oxygen diffuses (moves) into the blood and the carbon dioxide diffuses into the lungs. When providing inhalation sedation is added nitrous oxide into the respiratory system and as the blood does not contain any nitrous oxide it will diffuse across the alveolar membrane into the blood. It is then carried throughout the body with it acting upon the brain within 3–5 minutes. The same process occurs as it enters the fat, muscles and connective tissue. The patient remains sedated, because the supply of nitrous oxide to the lungs and then into the body is continual until the machine is switched off. Due to the inhalation sedation mode of action any change in the concentration of nitrous oxide being administered means that time should be allowed for the altered effect to take place, coupled with, upon termination of the gases, the patient's recovery should not be impeded, because all the nitrous oxide is exhaled [1].

Elimination from the body

Nitrous oxide is eliminated through exhalation with 99% removed almost as soon as delivery is stopped. The remaining 1% is eliminated through the skin and lungs over the next 24 hours. If a patient is not administered 100% oxygen for 3–5 minutes at the end of the procedure they will experience diffusion hypoxia:

- Stopping nitrous oxide will result in its elimination from the blood very quickly. This will result in more carbon dioxide than usual being expelled together with the nitrous oxide. This reduces the amount of carbon dioxide in the blood. The reason a breath is taken is attributed to the rising level of carbon dioxide in the blood. If the level is reduced the patient will not breathe and will suffer respiratory depression. This is known as the second gas effect.
- When the inhalation sedation machine is switched off nitrous oxide will leave the blood and flood into the lungs to be exhaled, because the concentration in the blood is higher than that in the lungs. This will result in a dilution of the oxygen levels within the lungs and the patient will experience hypoxia, headaches, nausea and lethargy [1].

The stages and planes of anaesthesia

When discussing the effects that patients experience when receiving inhalation sedation the planes of anaesthesia are used (Figure 5.10). There are four stages to the planes of anaesthesia with some being divided further. For patient co-operation the provision of inhalation sedation should be delivered in plane 1 or 2 of stage 1. This is because most patients while being sedated move gradually from one plane to another in respect of the feelings and experiences they

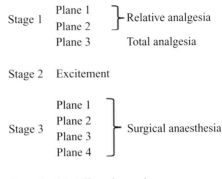

Stage 2   Excitement

Stage 4   Medullary depression

Figure 5.10 Planes of anaesthesia.

encounter without adverse effects. Plane 3 is on the threshold of stage 2 (excitement stage) and therefore provides a wider margin of safety, because if stage 2 was achieved it would provide light anaesthesia. This would be dangerous/unsafe and is contraindicative of its use. Any depth of general anaesthesia is not to be countenanced unless the clinical environment is correct. It is imperative in order to avoid over sedation to monitor a patient's response to the percentage of nitrous oxide being administered, because of the over lap in percentages and the different subjective experiences a patient will encounter. It is also important to remember that patients are individuals and that the percentage of nitrous oxide required will be variable [1,10].

Subjective experiences felt by patients

Stage 1
This stage is sometimes referred to as the induction stage. This is the time between the first administration of drugs and the loss of consciousness. Patients are conscious and able to communicate. They feel disorientated, experience analgesia and their respiration may be irregular. This stage is known as the analgesia stage and is divided into 3 planes [1,10]:

   Plane 1: Moderate sedation and analgesia. The patient is administered between 5% and 25% nitrous oxide. The clinical effects experienced by a patient are as follows: They feel more relaxed, which leads to a reduction of anxiety, consequently placing no unnecessary physiological stress on the heart. Their perception to painful stimuli is reduced and they experience some tingling sensations in their fingers, toes, lips and tongue. There may be minor amnesic effects due to the nitrous oxide. Patients at this stage can be communicative, able to answer any questions and are responsive to requests.

   Plane 2: Dissociation sedation and analgesia. The patient is administered between 20% and 55% nitrous oxide. The clinical effects experienced by

TYPES OF SEDATION

a patient are as follows: They feel further relaxed and appear unperturbed by the dental environment. They feel detached from their surroundings. Their fears and anxieties have disappeared and their perception to painful stimuli has been further reduced. They feel they are floating, euphoric, lethargic and very contented. They very rarely feel nauseous. When responding to questions they will be slow to respond and their voice will be husky and sluggish. The patient is able to maintain an open mouth. The ability to keep their mouth open is vital and if they cannot it is an indication that they are over sedated. A mouth prop must never be used. At this point the percentage of nitrous oxide would have to be lessened to reduce the depth of sedation. The amnesic effect of nitrous oxide is slightly more at this stage.

Plane 3: Total amnesia. The patient is administered between 50% and 70% nitrous oxide. The clinical effects experienced by a patient are as follows: Their fears and anxieties are eliminated, as is their response to pain. Although the amnesic effect of nitrous oxide is apparent the patient can become agitated, have a fixed stare and have unpleasant hallucinatory dreams. They may also feel nauseous and their mouth may close. If these responses to inhalation sedation occur it can be impossible to undertake the patient's treatment, as the sedation is too deep for them. In this circumstance the nitrous oxide should be reduced by 10% to remove these experiences. The reduction will reduce the effects and the patient will once again be cooperative and conducive to treatment.

Stage 2

This is known as the excitement stage. The patient will lose consciousness and may make uncontrolled movements, vomit, hold their breath and their pupils may become dilated. Their heart rate and breathing is irregular. This, coupled with potential vomit, may result in the airway being compromised [1,10].

Stage 3

This is the surgical stage. All the patient's muscles relax with their breathing returning to a regular rhythm. Their eye movements slow and then stop, becoming fixed with a central stare. This stage has been divided into four planes, where the following will be observed:

- The eyes roll and then become fixed.
- The corneal and laryngeal reflexes are lost.
- Reflexes are lost and the pupils dilate.
- The intercostal muscles become paralysed, abdominal respiration is shallow and the pupils are dilated [1,10].

Stage 4

This is also referred to as the overdose stage, as the patient will have been administered too high a percentage of drug resulting in medullary depression. Their breathing stops and a potential cardiovascular collapse ensues. This should not occur and would require immediate action to provide the patient with respiratory and cardiovascular support [1,10].

Patient management and the provision of inhalation sedation

When undertaking treatment using inhalation sedation, the aim should be to use a quiet environment and provide the patient with as little nitrous oxide as possible, coupled with hypnotic suggestion. The patient's sedation level should be kept in plane 1 or 2 of stage 1 of the stages of anaesthesia. Good patient management is important to assess the patient's problems, fears and worries before, during and after treatment. The team must have a confident and sympathetic approach and be able to calm the patient's fears and concerns in order to build their confidence in not only the team, but also the technique. Trust will be gained and a rapport built. Good communication is important. To achieve this, time must be taken to explain the sedation technique, its effectiveness and that it is a safe mode of sedation. The patient must be allowed to ask questions about their appointment. He/she must be able to ascertain that the team believe in the sedation they are providing and they have to feel relaxed, otherwise the sedation could be ineffective. When communicating with patients the team should talk in a soothing, calm voice. They must also give praise and encouragement using plain language, so that the patient fully understands what is happening from the beginning to the end of their appointment. Once the patient is recovered, it is advantageous to evaluate the session with the patient so that cooperation may improve at the next appointment [1].

Preparation for a patient's dental appointment

The team must prepare for the patient's appointments so that safe sedation is provided in a suitable environment. All the required dental instruments, material and medicaments must be available for the procedure, with the patient's notes, consent form and radiographs being present. All emergency equipment must be checked and be readily available. The team may choose to inform the receptionist that they do not wish to receive any interruptions during the treatment session and to divert any telephone calls to another surgery, warning other colleagues not to enter. Adequate ventilation is important and staff should be rotated, ensuring that the same personnel do not work with patients receiving inhalation sedation for long periods. If there is limited qualified staff to deliver this form of sedation, then the appointments should be spread over the working week to avoid continual exposure to nitrous oxide, as it can have

TYPES OF SEDATION

adverse effects on health. Different size masks must be available to ensure that the patient has a good fitting one. If the patient has had an acclimatisation appointment they will have already been measured for one and hopefully will bring it on the day of their appointment. Whether the machine is a piped system or a mobile one, it must be checked prior to use. This pre-check ensures that it is safe and in the case of the mobile machine there are enough gases for the procedure to avoid the disruption of changing a cylinder. When undertaking this check it must be remembered not to grease or oil any of the connections [1].

Checking a piped inhalation sedation machine

- Place the white oxygen pipe into the oxygen outlet valve (Figure 5.11) making sure that it is secure.
- Place the blue nitrous oxide pipe into the nitrous oxide outlet valve (Figure 5.12) making sure that it is secure.
- Connect the scavenging system ready to be used at the start of the procedure.
- Turn the dial on the delivery head to 100% oxygen (Figure 5.13).
- Turn the ON button (Figure 5.14) and keep turning until the metal ball in the oxygen flow meter reaches 8L/min (Figure 5.15).
- Alter the oxygen flow to 50%. This will automatically dial in 50% nitrous oxide and the metal ball in the nitrous oxide flow meter will rise to 4L/min (Figure 5.16, centre). The metal ball in the oxygen flow meter will drop to 4. This will allow the calibration of the machine to be checked. The metal balls in both flow meters should be level (Figure 5.16, left and right) indicating that the gases being delivered to a patient will be accurate.
- The nitrous oxide safety cut out valve must be checked to ensure that if delivery of oxygen stops the nitrous oxide would automatically cut off. This prevents the delivery of pure nitrous oxide, which if not noticed will result

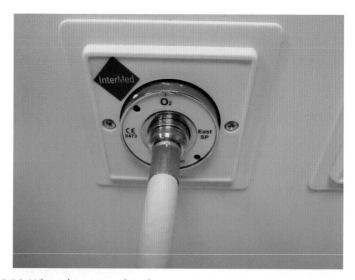

Figure 5.11 White tubing into outlet valve.

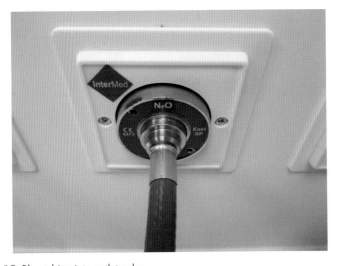

Figure 5.12 Blue tubing into outlet valve.

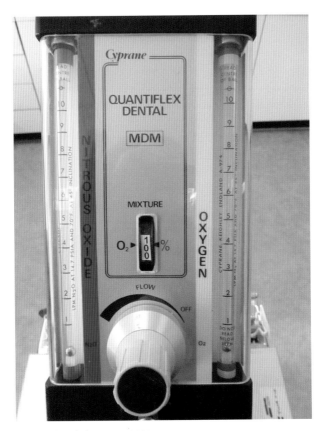

Figure 5.13 Delivery head showing 100% oxygen.

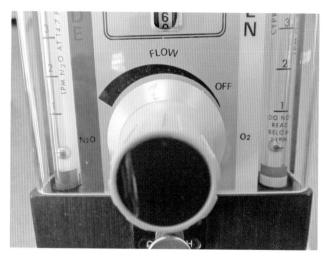

Figure 5.14 ON button.

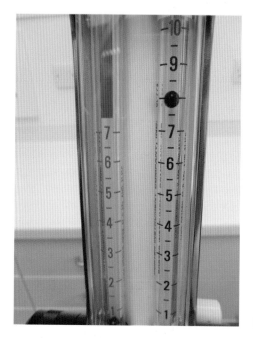

Figure 5.15 Oxygen at 8L/min.

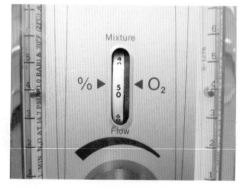

Figure 5.16 Dial at 50% oxygen and nitrous oxide (centre) and calibrated balls at 4L/min for both gases (left and right).

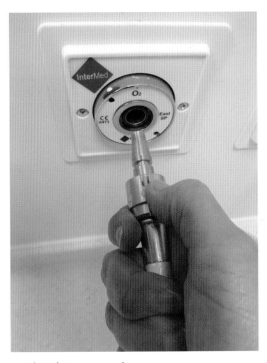

Figure 5.17 Oxygen tubing being removed.

in death. This check is undertaken by simulating oxygen failure by removing the oxygen piping from the outlet valve (Figure 5.17). If functional, the nitrous oxide will stop delivery and both metal balls in the flow meters will drop to zero (Figures 5.18a and b). The oxygen pipe is replaced into the outlet valve, the flow meter returned to 100% and the machine switched off.

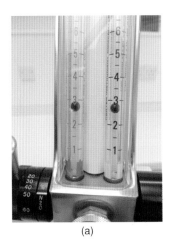
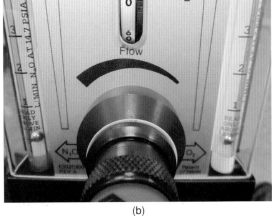

(a)   (b)

Figure 5.18 Balls in flow meter dropping (a) and dropped to zero (b).

TYPES OF SEDATION

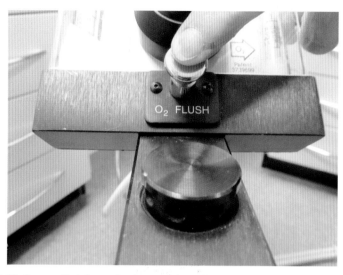

Figure 5.19 Oxygen flush button being pressed.

- The oxygen flush button is pressed (Figure 5.19) to ensure that it is functional and to inflate the reservoir bag (Figure 5.20) so that it can be checked for any leaks or holes. The weakest part of the reservoir bag is the neck where it is placed onto the machine. The reservoir bag must be removed to check that the air entrainment valve is not blocked and then replaced. This is undertaken by placing a finger into it (Figure 5.21).

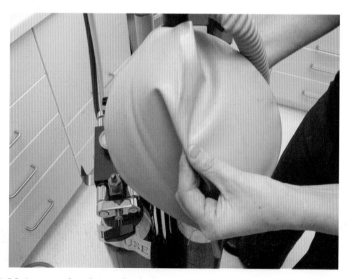

Figure 5.20 Reservoir bag being checked.

TYPES OF SEDATION

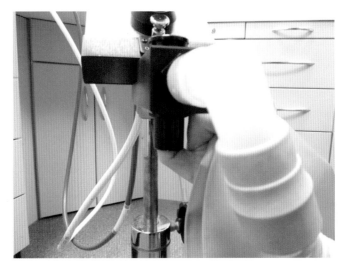

Figure 5.21 Reservoir bag removed and air entrainment valve being checked.

- The last check is to inspect all tubing for holes and that they have not perished (Figure 5.22).

Safety mechanisms of a piped inhalation sedation machine
- The nitrous oxide stops delivery if the oxygen supply fails.
- The reservoir bag allows monitoring of patient respiration.

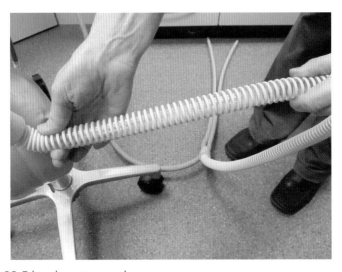

Figure 5.22 Tubing being inspected.

TYPES OF SEDATION

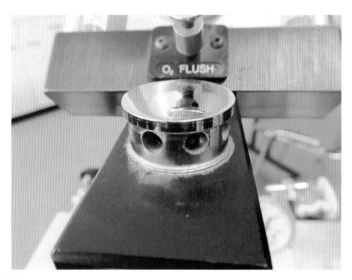

Figure 5.23 Air entrainment valve.

- The air entrainment valve (Figure 5.23) will allow atmospheric air to be inhaled if both gases stopped delivery.
- The scavenging system allows the excess waste nitrous oxide to be removed from the atmosphere.
- The flush button can be pressed if additional oxygen is required. When activated 30L/min of oxygen will be delivered to a patient.
- The machine will not allow any less than 30% oxygen to be delivered to a patient. This means that a patient cannot receive any more than 70% nitrous oxide, thus preventing them from entering stage 2, the excitement stage of the stages of anaesthesia, which is not an acceptable level.
- Different colour pipes.

Checking a mobile inhalation sedation machine

- All cylinders should be switched off and firmly fixed/tightened to the machine.
- There should be four cylinders attached. Two nitrous oxide (blue), one of which is in use (labelled) and the other is full (labelled). Two oxygen (black with a white collar), one is in use (labelled) and other is full (labelled). Labels to this effect must be attached (Figure 5.24).
- The blue piping is already connected to the nitrous oxide cylinder and white piping to the oxygen. This must be checked to ensure that it is correct (Figure 5.25).
- The full oxygen cylinder is firstly checked by turning the tap on to ensure that the oxygen gauge/dial reads full, which equates to approximately 2000 pounds per square inch (psi) (Figure 5.26). The tap must be turned off again.

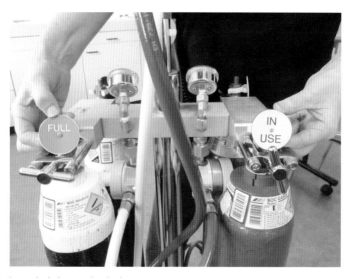

Figure 5.24 Labels being checked.

Depending upon the top of the oxygen cylinder the tap will either be opened by a key (Figure 5.27) or by hand.

- The oxygen flush button must be pressed to release all oxygen from the system and to check that it is functional. The dial indicator will return to zero. The reservoir bag will inflate and can be checked for leaks or tears. The weakest part of the bag is the neck. The reservoir bag must be removed to

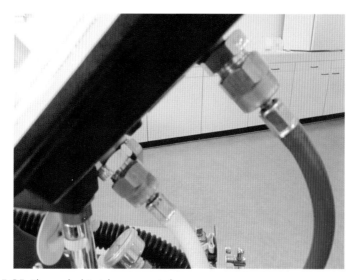

Figure 5.25 Blue and white tubes connected.

TYPES OF SEDATION

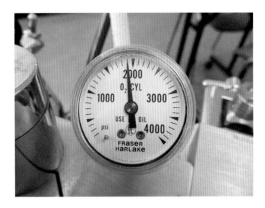

Figure 5.26 Oxygen dial showing approximately 2000psi.

check that the air entrainment valve is not blocked and then replaced. This is undertaken by placing a finger into it (Figure 5.21).

- The in-use oxygen cylinder is now checked by turning the tap on, making sure that it is at least a quarter full, which equates to 500psi. If the cylinder contains less than this a new cylinder must be fitted. As stock must be rotated, the existing full cylinder becomes the in-use one and the new cylinder will be the full one. When changing any cylinder it is important to ensure that the Bodok seal, similar to a washer (Figure 5.28) is not worn and is in place. This provides a seal between the cylinder and the machine, preventing leakage. The in-use cylinder is left switched on.
- The full nitrous oxide cylinder is switched on and off. The nitrous oxide gauge/dial will, if not recently used, reach 800psi. It is important to check

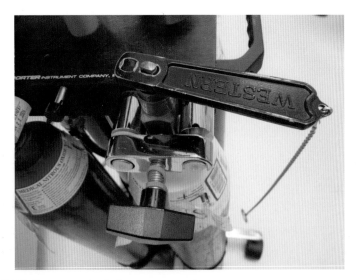

Figure 5.27 Key-operated cylinder.

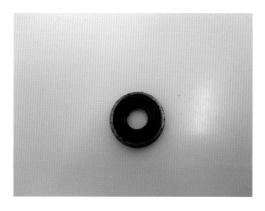

Figure 5.28 Bodok seal.

the type of the mobile relative analgesia machine being used because nitrous oxide in some machines cannot be flushed out of the system – therefore when switching on the in-use nitrous oxide cylinder it is impossible to tell how much it contains as its gauge/dial will still give the reading of the full cylinder. This is attributed to the nitrous oxide being a liquid under pressure. The gauge/dial will start to drop when most of the liquid has been used and the cylinder is nearly empty. It will start to change when the liquid turns to gas thus affecting the dial readings. A rough indication is to tap both cylinders while listening to the difference in sound. The duller the sound the less it contains. For more accuracy, the cylinders can be weighed:

- A full cylinder weighs approximately 8.8kg.
- An empty cylinder weighs approximately 5.4kg.
- Therefore the gas equates to approximately 3.4kg.
- All cylinders have a plastic collar (Figures 5.29a and b) that is stamped with information relating to its content, such as the name, batch number, expiry date and approximate weight.

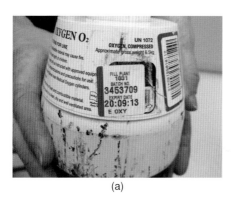

(a)

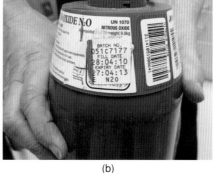

(b)

Figure 5.29 (a, b) Plastic sleeves on cylinders.

TYPES OF SEDATION

- The in-use nitrous oxide should be left switched on while checks are made.
- The automatic nitrous oxide safety cut-off valve is checked in the same way as the piped machine, by setting the flow meter to 8L/min of 100% oxygen, altering the percentage to 50% which alters the flow of nitrous oxide and oxygen to 4L/min each. This allows calibration of the machine to be checked at the same time. The in-use oxygen cylinder is switched off. As oxygen supply failure has been simulated the nitrous oxide should automatically fail and both metal balls in the flow meters should drop to zero after a slight delay. As the machine is mobile it will not have a continuous supply of gases, unlike the piped machine where the metal balls drop to zero instantly. This is attributed to a small amount of oxygen being left in the machine and the nitrous oxide will still deliver until all oxygen has dissipated. Once this check has been undertaken satisfactorily the in-use oxygen cylinder can be switched back on.
- The in-use nitrous oxide cylinder is then switched off.
- If a patient is ready for treatment and all tubing has been visually inspected, ensuring that they have not perished, holes are not present and the scavenging system is attached and switched on, the in-use oxygen cylinder will remain on, with the percentage dial being returned to 100%.
- If a patient is not present for treatment, then the in-use oxygen cylinder will be switched off. The oxygen flush button will be pressed to expel all oxygen from the machine with all tubing being inspected to ensure that they are not perished/damaged or holed [1].

Safety mechanisms of a mobile inhalation sedation machine

- The nitrous oxide stops delivery if the oxygen supply fails.
- The reservoir bag allows monitoring of a patient's respiration.
- The air entrainment valve (Figure 5.23) will allow atmospheric air to be inhaled if both gases fail to deliver.
- The scavenging system allows the excess waste nitrous oxide to be removed from the atmosphere.
- The flush button can be pressed if additional oxygen is required. When activated, 30L/min of oxygen will be delivered to a patient.
- The machine will not allow any less than 30% oxygen to be delivered to a patient. This means that a patient will not receive any more than 70% nitrous oxide, preventing them from entering stage 2, the excitement stage of the stages of anesthesia, which is not an acceptable level.
- Different colour pipes and connection nuts are stamped with either nitrous oxide or oxygen (Figure 5.30).
- In use, full and empty labels give an indication of the cylinder status. However, these should not be relied upon and the machine must be checked prior to use.

TYPES OF SEDATION

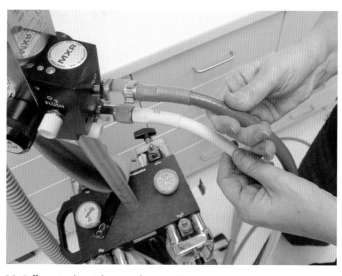

Figure 5.30 Different colour tubing and connection nuts.

- 'E' size cylinders have unique pin indexing (Figures 5.31a and b) which makes it impossible for the wrong cylinder to be connected to the machine.
- The Bodok seal, which provides a tight fit between the cylinder and the machine to prevent leakage [1].

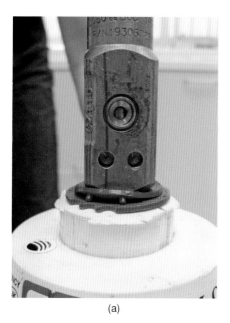
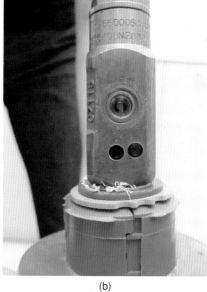

(a)   (b)

Figure 5.31 (a, b) Pin index system.

Delivery of inhalation sedation to a patient

The inhalation sedation machine is checked. The gases are switched on with the oxygen percentage being set at 100% and the scavenging system attached. Once the patient has had their medical history updated and any pre-medical checks undertaken, the clinician is happy that consent is still valid and the patient is content, the procedure with inhalation sedation will commence:

- The patient is reassured and invited to take a seat in the dental chair. The procedure is re-explained to them with any anxieties, doubts or fears allayed. Any questions are answered.
- If a nasal mask has not already been fitted, then a suitable size is selected and shown to the patient. They are asked to place it over their nose and it is checked to ensure that it is seated correctly.
- The clinician will briefly explain in a quiet hypnotic voice the sensations/feelings that the patient may experience as the dental chair is slowly lowered to the supine position.
- As the inhalation sedation machine is already switched on with the oxygen being at 100%, the flow rate is placed at 8L/min for an adult patient and 6L/min for a paediatric patient.
- The reservoir bag must be observed to ensure it fills.
- The mask on the patient's nose is checked again and the scavenging system is switched on.
- The patient is given time to relax and once settled the oxygen mixture control is turned to 85%, introducing 15% nitrous oxide. The reservoir bag must be monitored to ensure that the flow rate of gases provided is adequate. If the reservoir bag over-inflates (Figure 5.32), it would mean that the initial flow rate was too much for the patient. They would not be using it all and the flow rate should be reduced. If the reservoir bag is under-inflated (Figure 5.33) it would indicate that the patient requires a higher flow rate, as they are trying to obtain more from the machine than is being provided, so the flow rate should be increased.
- The patient should be continued to be spoken to in a soft, quiet, hypnotic manner, reminding them of how they will feel. It is also advantageous to give encouragement and praise. This will allow a couple of minutes for the nitrous oxide to take effect with the patient experiencing the symptoms of plane 1 of stage 1 anaesthesia.
- If there is no response to the small percentage of nitrous oxide being provided, then a further 5% should be administered, allowing time for it to take effect before providing more. If required further 5% incremental doses should be administered until 30% nitrous oxide is reached, remembering that all patients are individuals and therefore will require different amounts to provide them with adequate and safe sedation. At 30% nitrous oxide the patient will definitely be in plane 1 if not plane 2 of the stages of anaesthesia,

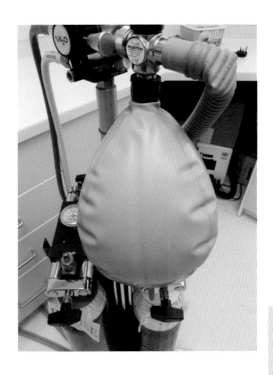

Figure 5.32 An over-inflated bag.

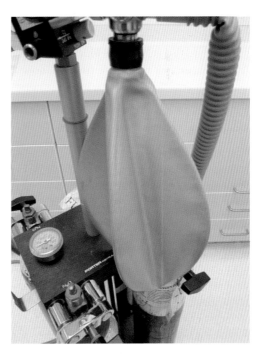

Figure 5.33 An under-inflated bag.

TYPES OF SEDATION

which is correct for inhalation sedation. It is at this stage that treatment can commence. If a patient has attended before, well written notes are invaluable, as they will inform the team of how much nitrous oxide the patient received during their last visit and if there were any complications.

- Depending upon the treatment it may be necessary for the patient to receive a local anaesthetic before the procedure is undertaken.
- When treatment is complete the nitrous oxide is slowly reduced until the patient is receiving 100% oxygen for 3–5 minutes to prevent diffusion hypoxia.
- The nasal mask should be removed before the inhalation machine and scavenging system are switched off.
- The patient is praised and asked to remain on the premises for a further 20–30 minutes to ensure that they are fit for discharge.
- When the patient has left, the surgery is restored and prepared for the next patient in the normal way with notes being updated.

Throughout the patient's appointment, vital signs are clinically monitored for signs of over sedation or distress, with any/all appropriate action being taken. Electrical monitoring is not essential, because the patient is receiving a minimum of 30% oxygen at all times. If a pulse oximeter was in use, its readings would reflect this and it would indicate that the patient was supplied with sufficient amounts of oxygen. They must be continually encouraged and reassured, so that they feel safe and secure, thus cooperative. It must be remembered that all clinicians administer inhalation sedation in a different manner as patient requirements are individual and their experience with its use will vary [1].

The gases used during the delivery of inhalation sedation

Nitrous oxide

Joseph Priestley produced nitrous oxide in 1772 and it was then researched by Humphry Davy. He introduced it as a recreational drug to the upper classes in 1799, where it was used at parties for the amusement of on-lookers. The user would giggle, have slurred speech, stumble and fall down. It was some 36 years later that it was used for medical purposes. Dr. Horace Wells, an American dentist, recognised the effects of nitrous oxide in 1844. He volunteered to have a tooth extracted by his associate with its use. As he didn't experience any pain he introduced it to his patients. In the early stages inhalation sedation was very unpredictable due to lack of knowledge of its action. However, today's clinicians are aware of its clinical effects and can administer it quite safely. Nitrous oxide, when produced by the manufacturer, is compressed at 800psi to a liquid with its vapour being on top. As liquid is not as easily compressed

TYPES OF SEDATION

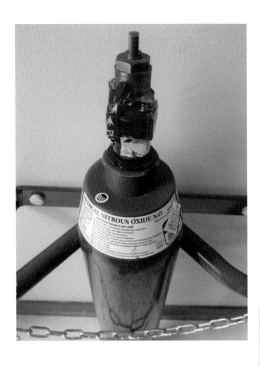

Figure 5.34 Nitrous oxide cylinder.

as gas the cylinder will only be partly full. It is supplied in cylinders which are blue (Figure 5.34). It doesn't cause irritation to the respiratory system but will depress the central nervous system and if used at 80% will lead to unconsciousness, despite it being a weak anaesthetic. Nitrous oxide can be toxic to the team if exposed to it for long periods, especially where a scavenging system is not in use and ventilation is inadequate [1,2].

Nitrous oxide toxicity

As nitrous oxide is minimally metabolised when exhaled by the patient it retains its potency. If the team use inhalation sedation regularly and/or for long periods, frequently, they will naturally be exposed to nitrous oxide. They will inhale it, especially if ventilation is poor and/or a scavenging system is not used. Nitrous oxide is toxic and can:

- decrease mental performance;
- inhibit the bone marrow function;
- cause infertility in female workers;
- lead to numbness in the peripheral extremities which can give a sensation of pins and needles;
- affect the vitamin B12 which is required for the brain and nervous system to function normally and is also required for blood to form;
- affect manual dexterity;

- cause anaemia;
- cause birth defects [1,2].

Control of Substances Hazardous to Health (COSHH) and nitrous oxide

COSHH ensures that the working environment for the team is safe. Employers must undertake risk assessments where any work involves exposure to hazardous substances. This allows the risks to health to be established and to implement any necessary precautions to reduce that risk, or where this is impossible to adequately control them. As nitrous oxide is an anaesthetic gas it is considered hazardous, as the benefit of its use is to the patient only. Therefore the exposure level must be reduced so that staff exposed to it suffer no adverse effects. The Health and Safety Commission have established Workplace Exposure Limits (WELs). The limits set are intended to prevent excessive exposure to named substances, thus limiting risk to health. The long-term exposure for nitrous oxide is a time-weighted average of 100 parts per million over an 8-hour period in any 24 hours. This allows for shift workers. Short-term exposure limits to nitrous oxide are not included [1,2,4].

Additional control measures

- Servicing by the manufacturer or authorised personnel will ensure that the machine is functioning correctly.
- Check the machine prior to use for leaks.
- Use of good fitting masks to prevent leakage.
- Good room ventilation. Any fans used must be placed on the floor, as nitrous oxide is heavier than air and collects at floor level.
- Limit the amount of sessions per week.
- Rotating staff so that they are not working with nitrous oxide on a regular basis.
- Encourage the patient not to talk to avoid any unnecessary nitrous oxide being exhaled into the room.
- Use of rubber dam to avoid exhalation of nitrous oxide into the room.
- Use of high volume aspiration to suction exhaled nitrous oxide.
- Air and personal nitrous oxide monitors to ensure that time-weighted averages are not exceeded.
- Anaesthetic gas scavenging systems. These attach to the inhalation sedation machine to remove the waste nitrous oxide from the surgery. There are two systems used: (1) an active system, which pumps the gases away, and (2) a passive system, which has one entry and one exit for the gas [1,4].

Oxygen

The use of oxygen when providing inhalation sedation is mandatory, as it is essential for life. It is a clear, colourless and odourless gas supplied in cylinders which are painted black with a white collar (Figure 5.35) and under pressure

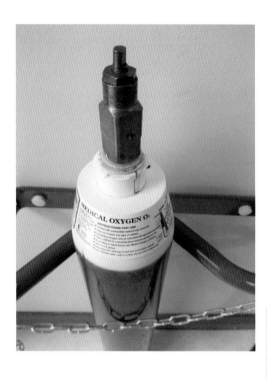

Figure 5.35 Oxygen cylinder.

at 2000psi. The connections, valves or fitments must never be lubricated with oil or grease as there is a danger of explosion. Oxygen is not flammable but will support combustion [1,2].

Some contraindications of usage

Certain dental procedures

Anterior dental treatment within the maxilla may prove difficult as the mask could prove to be a nuisance, especially in surgical procedures such as an apicectomy, where a flap once raised must be retracted.

A cold or flu

If the nose is blocked it makes it difficult to breathe and breathing by mouth is inevitable – therefore the inhalation sedation will be ineffective. Gases at a positive pressure may push any infection further into the respiratory system (dealt with previously within this chapter) [1].

Nasal obstruction

Patients who have large adenoids and tonsils make inhalation sedation difficult due to the obstruction/blockage of their nasal passages within the respiratory structure. For inhalation sedation to be effective patients must be able to breathe through their nasal passages and have a clear route to the lungs [1].

TYPES OF SEDATION

Claustrophobia

If a patient experiences claustrophobia in certain circumstances they may not be able to tolerate a nasal mask.

Tuberculosis and other acute pulmonary conditions

Prior to providing inhalation sedation the clinician may decide to contact the patient's doctor, because although nitrous oxide is not very irritant, it is more irritating than atmospheric air and it could irritate and exacerbate the patient's existing condition [1].

The psychiatric patient

Inhalation sedation changes patients' perception of things and makes them feel detached from their surroundings. This may not be beneficial to patients whose emotional state is reliant upon medication as this change may upset them. The clinician may decide to contact the patient's doctor or psychiatrist to establish if this mode of sedation would be suitable [1].

Immunosuppressed patients

Nitrous oxide affects the production and function of the white blood cells whose action is to fight infection and remove dead and injured tissue. Immunosuppressed patients are more at risk of post-operative infections. This is attributed to their white blood cells not being as effective as those of a person who is not immunosuppressed. Consequently, they are not able to overcome infections as easily. If nitrous oxide is used it will lower the production and the function of their white blood cells, further delaying their recovery.

Pregnancy

Inhalation sedation should be avoided in the first trimester of known pregnancy, because the effect of nitrous oxide could cause a spontaneous abortion. It should be restricted to the second and third trimesters. Fetal blood contains 50% of that of the mother – therefore nitrous oxide will pass the placental barrier affecting the DNA production and could result in birth defects. A pre-mix of 50% nitrous oxide and 50% oxygen is used for pain relief within childbirth and is known as entonox [1].

Myasthenia gravis

This is an uncommon chronic, autoimmune disease that causes muscle weakness and excessive muscle tiredness. The use of nitrous oxide will potentially increase muscle weakness [1].

Pneumothorax, middle ear and sinus disease

Nitrous oxide can enter areas within the body faster than the existing nitrogen can leave. This could lead to a short-term increase in volume within the gut, middle ear etc. and in rare cases increased harmful effects can result, such as a pneumothorax [13].

ORAL SEDATION

This is the lightest form of sedation offered to patients for treatment. Prescribing can be by the clinician or the patient's doctor. When a prescription is provided the patient can only obtain enough of the drug for the impending treatment session. They are used to relieve fear and reduce anxiety prior to their dental appointment and are taken orally either in a liquid or a tablet form. Oral sedation works well for most patients allowing them to relax, with some having little or no memory of their treatment. This mode of sedation can involve the patient taking the medication at home, at the surgery or a combination of the two. The common drugs used belong to the family of drugs known as benzo-diazepines. Their action and elimination on and within the body is the same as for intravenous sedation. This means that patient care, in respect of assessment and monitoring, coupled with the pre and post-operative instructions attached to intravenous sedation will be identical for patients receiving oral sedation. Well kept records are important as these will highlight the effects of previous doses received, which means that dosage can be adjusted to suit the patient's previous response [1].

Advantages of oral sedation

The advantages of oral sedation are:

- Easy to administer, as only a small tablet or spoonful of medicine is taken.
- Accepted by most people due to this mode of sedation being likened to taking routine medication.
- Produces sedation, relaxes patients and provides some amnesic effects.
- A cannula is not always placed, so ideal for needle phobics.
- Specialised training is not always required as with intravenous and inhalation sedation, as it is safe and easy to monitor.
- Decreased incidence and severity of adverse drug reactions.
- Not expensive to provide.
- Works well for most patients [1].

Disadvantages of oral sedation

The disadvantages of oral sedation are:

- If the patient is given the medication to take at home they are being trusted to take it as directed.
- The patient must be able to comply with rigid pre and post-operative in-structions. Concerns arising: If the patient has been given the medication for home use are driving to the surgery and not bringing an escort. The

TYPES OF SEDATION

clinician is putting their trust in the patient to comply with these and other instructions.

- Unless a cannula is placed there is no venous access.
- A patient could attend their appointment over sedated.
- The drug cannot be titrated against patient response – therefore the depth of sedation cannot be altered.
- The drug used does not provide any analgesia.
- The drug can take some time to take effect.
- The drug used stays in the body for a long time.
- Absorption and elimination of the drug can be erratic [1,5].

Drugs commonly used in oral sedation

Diazepam (valium)

It is a benzodiazepine derivative which is commonly used for treating conditions such as anxiety, insomnia, seizures, and muscle spasms. It is also used prior to surgical procedures to reduce tension and anxiety that could be related to the impending procedure. It results in sedation, has anxiolytic, anticonvulsant, hypnotic, muscle relaxant and amnesic properties, with these being reversed by flumazenil should the need arise. It can take between 30 minutes and an hour to take effect after administration. The precise dose for each patient is difficult to calculate, as the amount prescribed is weight related and it has a long half-life of approximately 36–57 hours [1].

Diazepam presentation

- 2mg (white tablet)
- 5mg (yellow tablet)
- 10mg (blue tablet)
- Diazepam syrup, 2mg/5ml and 5mg/5ml [1]

Usual dose prescribed

- For an adult 10mg can be given 1 hour before the procedure or 5mg the night before, 5mg upon wakening and 5mg 2 hours prior to the procedure [1,5].
- For children, half the adult dose is prescribed [1].
- For elderly patients, half the adult dose is prescribed, although some patients may require a higher dose than for children [1].

Some contraindications of usage

Children

Under the age of 10 years a child's response/reaction to the drug can be unpredictable. Some children may become excitable and unmanageable.

The elderly

They will be more sensitive to diazepam and the elimination from the body may be prolonged.

Patients prescribed anti-depressants

These drugs can enhance the effects of diazepam.

Pregnancy

The effects of diazepam could harm the fetus [5].

Alcoholics

The effects of diazepam will be enhanced by alcohol [5].

Myasthenia gravis

Diazepam is a muscle relaxant, which could further weaken the patient's muscles.

Allergy or sensitivity to benzodiazepines

If taken the patient will suffer an allergic reaction which could be life threatening [5].

Antihistamines

Drowsiness may be increased due to antihistamines. Despite being primarily prescribed for allergies, some sedation is produced as a side effect [5].

Temazepam

Temazepam is a controlled drug belonging to the family of benzodiazepines. It is generally provided to patients who have difficult sleep patterns. It produces sedation and a state of relaxation. It has anxiolytic, anticonvulsant, muscle relaxant properties and is considered to be a hypnotic drug. Its action is reversed by flumazenil should the need arise. It is more expensive than diazepam, but is more effective with a much shorter half-life of 8–10 hours, which makes it an ideal pre-medication, especially if it is to be used in conjunction with intravenous agents. Like diazepam the dose prescribed is weight related [1].

Temazepam presentation

- 10mg (white tablet)
- 20mg (white tablet)
- 10mg per 5ml elixir [1]

Usual dose prescribed

- For an adult the usual dose is 10–30mg 1 hour prior to procedure [1,5].
- For children, half the adult dose [1].
- For elderly patients, half the adult dose is prescribed although some patients may require a higher dose than for children [1].

Some contraindications of usage

Children

Under the age of 10 years, a child's response/reaction to the drug can be unpredictable. Some children may become excitable and unmanageable.

The elderly

They will be more sensitive to temazepam and the elimination from the body may be prolonged.

Patients prescribed anti-depressants

These drugs can enhance the effects of temazepam.

Pregnancy

The effects of temazepam could harm the fetus [5].

Alcoholics

The effects of temazepam will be enhanced by alcohol [5].

Myasthenia gravis

Temazepam is a muscle relaxant, which could further weaken the patient's muscles.

Allergy or sensitivity to benzodiazepines

If taken, the patient will suffer an allergic reaction which could be life-threatening [1].

Antihistamines

Drowsiness may be increased due to antihistamines. Despite being primarily prescribed for allergies, some sedation is produced as a side effect [5].

Factors/precautions/considerations when prescribing

The best environment for the patient to take the medication and optimum time for it to be taken

- If in the patient's home the clinician has to be sure that the patient will take the medication as directed.
- They will reach the surgery safely with an escort.
- Will attend the appointment [1].

Pre and post-operative instructions

The patient must be able to comply with the rigid pre and post-operative instructions. If they cannot, then oral sedation is not prescribed [1].

Usage with another drug

If intravenous sedation is being used in conjunction with oral sedation a reduced intravenous dose will be required. Slow titration of the drug will avoid over sedation. The dose already received cannot be altered and the absorption is unknown [1].

Experience of the dental team

The knowledge and skills of the team providing the oral sedation will ensure that the patient is treated safely.

BIBLIOGRAPHY

1. Hospital Course notes.
2. en.wikipedia.org/wiki/Midazolam
3. drugs.emedtv.com/midazolam/midazolam.html
4. http://www.hse.gov.uk/coshh/table1.pdf
5. www.dentalfearcentral.org/oral_sedation.html
6. en.wikipedia.org/wiki/Flumazenil
7. General Dental Council Standards Guidance document.
8. Department of Health, Conscious sedation in the provision of dental care, www.dh.gov.uk
9. en.wikipedia.org/wiki/Propofol
10. en.wikipedia.org/wiki/Guedal's_classification
11. en.wikipedia.org/wiki/Nitrous Oxide
12. en.wikipedia.org/wiki/Oxygen
13. www.frca.co.uk/article.aspx?articlead=100358

TYPES OF SEDATION

Chapter 6
Medical emergencies

LEARNING OUTCOMES

At the end of this chapter you will have a clear understanding of:

- Recognising the signs and symptoms of common emergencies that could occur in the dental surgery.
- Managing these conditions efficiently.
- Reducing the risk of an emergency in the surgery.

INTRODUCTION

Any patient could suffer an emergency while undergoing treatment in the surgery. Life threatening emergencies are rare, but they can happen and the team must be prepared to manage any condition that occurs. For the team to be able to manage any and all emergencies they must seek the appropriate training in medical emergencies and resuscitation. A dental practice can, in conjunction with training, implement various mechanisms to reduce the risk of an emergency, which is naturally preferable to having to deal with one [1].

PREVENTION OF MEDICAL EMERGENCIES

Prevention is much better than having to deal with a patient who is experiencing an emergency, as it is stressful and disturbing not only for the patient but also for the team, even if the patient does make a full recovery. To reduce the risk of

---

Basic Guide to Dental Sedation Nursing, First Edition. Nicola Rogers.
© 2011 Nicola Rogers. Published 2011 by Blackwell Publishing Ltd.

an emergency within the surgery the following points should be implemented as they are deemed to be good practice [1]:

- All staff, including the receptionist, should undertake regular training and attend updates in emergency situations and resuscitation to ensure that their knowledge and skills are in line with the current resuscitation council (UK) guidelines.
- Medical emergency simulations are extremely valuable as they allow the team to implement their knowledge and practice their skills in a controlled environment without compromising a patient's health. When undertaken, all participants should discuss the activity to establish if the simulation went well and if not how it could be improved should it ever occur in a real-life situation.
- All staff should understand their role during an emergency. The normal situation is for the nurse to obtain the emergency drugs/equipment and to assist the clinician as directed, while the receptionist alerts the emergency services. However, if the nurse is the first person on the scene, then he/she should administer first-line treatment to the patient and give clear instructions to others while waiting for the dentist and/or the emergency services arrival so that the patient's condition hopefully remains stable.
- Careful assessment and good patient management can prevent emergencies. Updating a patient's medical history every time they visit the dental practice would establish if there has been any change in their condition or medication since their last visit. All the team should be encouraged to look at a patient's medical history to make themselves aware of any condition/s that the patient may suffer. In this way they can prepare for any eventuality and plan how they would assist the clinician to facilitate the patient's recovery. If a dental nurse is aware of a patient's medical condition they can request that the patient places their medication on the work surface for easy access. By taking/updating a medical history from a patient a clinician can establish the patient's medical fitness. They can evaluate the information discussed and decide whether the patient would be better managed within a hospital setting. The method commonly used is the American Society of Anaesthesiologists' (ASA's) classification of medical fitness as explained in Chapter 4.
- It is imperative to monitor the patient's vital signs during and after treatment, with monitoring commencing as soon as they enter the practice, with any concerns being relayed to the clinician.
- Emergency drugs and equipment should be easily accessible. A daily check should be undertaken to ensure that all drugs are in date and that emergency equipment is functional. Any drugs due to expire must be ordered immediately, with any that are out of date being replaced. These checks should be fully documented to avoid any confusion which could lead to a serious failure. All emergency equipment must be serviced at recommended intervals

with all documentation being kept. All staff should be aware of the contents of the emergency drugs box and know which medication is used for any/each arising condition. Audits of these activities should take place on a regular basis.

- Recording any incidents in the patient's notes is a reminder to yourself and is informative to others who may treat the patient in the future so that you and they can be prepared for the eventuality should it reoccur.
- Postponing treatment should be considered if it is identified that the patient is unwell, allowing him or her time to recover and, if needed, seek the necessary appropriate medical attention.
- Scheduling appointments to suit the patient's medical condition can help to prevent problems occurring. For example, if a patient is diabetic (type 1 or 2) then an appointment just after a meal is preferable as they will have eaten and their blood sugar would not be low, thereby decreasing the risk of them experiencing a hypoglycaemic episode.
- Risk assessments to look at the ergonomics of the practice to establish any difficulties you might encounter should an emergency arise.

LEGAL ASPECTS DEALING WITH MEDICAL EMERGENCIES

Dental professionals have a duty of care to patients and are expected to deal with any emergency that occurs in the surgery. The implication of any action taken irrespective of the outcome doesn't mean that they were negligent.

DEALING WITH MEDICAL EMERGENCIES

Two mistakes are most common in the management of emergencies. The first is to attempt to do too much and the second doing too little – therefore team effort is important. This ensures that everything that could possibly be done to aid patient recovery is carried out and that nothing is missed [1].

Control of medical emergencies

- When an emergency occurs in the surgery the team need to assess their surroundings to ensure not only the patient's safety, but also their own, because if they injure themselves they will not be able to aid the patient. This is a common mistake which could lead to unnecessary accidents occurring due to the team being in familiar surroundings and possibly forgetting to check for hazards [1].

MEDICAL EMERGENCIES

- The patient's general condition and vital signs should be assessed to determine the preliminary diagnosis, which is not always the definitive one. Continual monitoring is essential to recognise any changes in the patient's medical status, which can then be acted upon accordingly. It is important to check for any injuries that the patient may have sustained so that first aid can be administered promptly. Should an injury occur the team should prioritise and deal with whichever is more life threatening [1].
- Whenever a patient collapses and it is realised that an emergency has occurred help should always be called for. You should never attempt to cope on your own, because help that could possibly be more experienced could take the lead and request that you support them as they direct or if this is not the case take instructions from you. For example, they could call the emergency services and fetch the appropriate drugs, oxygen and masks [1].

Emergency drugs box and equipment

For a dental practice to manage the emergencies that can occur in the surgery they should have an easily identifiable area/box/trolley housing the recommended drugs and equipment required [1].

Drugs
- Adrenaline (1:1000 1mg/ml) (Figure 6.1)
- Aspirin, dispersible (300mg) (Figure 6.2)
- Glucagon (1mg) (Figure 6.3)
- Glyceryl trinitrate (GTN) spray (400mcg per dose) (Figure 6.4)

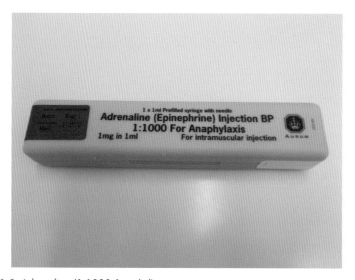

Figure 6.1 Adrenaline (1:1000 1mg/ml).

MEDICAL EMERGENCIES

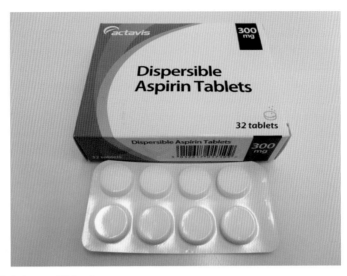

Figure 6.2 Aspirin (300mg).

- Midazolam (5mg/ml or 10mg/ml, buccal or intranasal)
- Oral glucose/tablets/gel/powder (Figure 6.5)
- Oxygen (D size with a pressure reduction valve and flow meter) (Figure 6.6)
- Salbutamol (100mcg per dose) (Figure 6.7) [1,8]

Where possible any drugs in a solution should be drawn into a pre-filled syringe, saving time and making them easier to administer. As intramuscular,

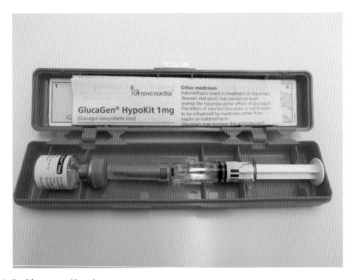

Figure 6.3 Glucagon (1mg).

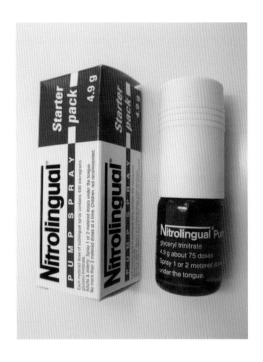

Figure 6.4 Glyceryl trinitrate spray
(400mcg per dose).

inhalation, sublingual, buccal and nasal routes of drug administration are faster
in an emergency they should be the preferred routes to use, with the intravenous
route of drugs being discouraged within a general practice setting. Portable
oxygen cylinders should be of a suitable size to enable them to be carried,
as well as containing sufficient oxygen to allow enough oxygen delivery to

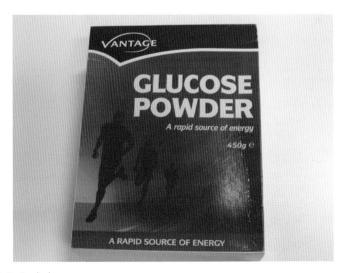

Figure 6.5 Oral glucose.

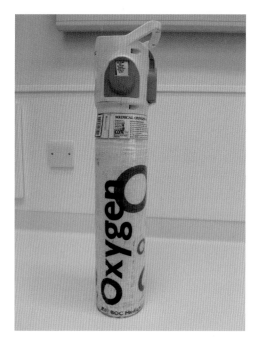

Figure 6.6 CD size oxygen cylinder.

patients at an adequate flow rate, for example 10–15L/min, until the arrival of the emergency services or until the patient fully recovers. A full 'D' size oxygen cylinder contains 340L of oxygen and if administered to a patient at a flow rate of 10–15L/min it will provide up to 20–30 minutes of oxygen. It may be

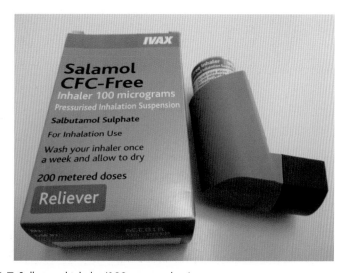

Figure 6.7 Salbutamol inhaler (100mcg per dose).

MEDICAL EMERGENCIES

necessary to have two cylinders within the practice to ensure that the supply of oxygen does not fail when it is used during an emergency [1].

Equipment
Where possible all emergency medical equipment within the practice should be latex free and single use only [1]:

- Different size oxygen face masks with tubing.
- Size 1, 2, 3 and 4 oropharyngeal airways (Figure 6.8).
- Pocket mask with an oxygen port (Figure 6.9).
- A self-inflating bag and mask with an oxygen reservoir bag and tubing (Figure 6.10) with different size masks to accommodate both paediatric and adult patients. If staff members have been appropriately trained to use them a 1L bag should be stocked.
- Portable suction (Figure 6.11) with suction catheters and tubing. A Yankauer sucker (Figure 6.12) would be an ideal suction tip to hold.
- Different size, single-use sterile syringes and needles (Figure 6.13).
- A large volume spacer device for inhaled bronchodilators (Figure 6.14).
- A blood glucose monitoring measurement kit (Figure 6.15).
- Automated external defibrillator (AED) (Figure 6.16).

AEDs are expected to be available in a dental practice as they require very little training to use them safely and they reduce mortality rates from cardiac arrest. All staff should be familiar with the device they have in their practice and they do not have to be trained to use one. However, training will increase the effectiveness of its use, improving the speed at which the pads are placed

MEDICAL EMERGENCIES

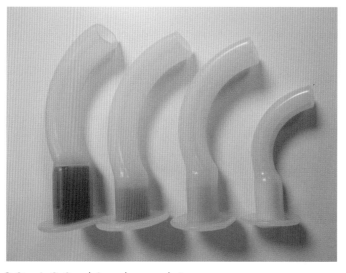

Figure 6.8 Size 1, 2, 3 and 4 oropharyngeal airways.

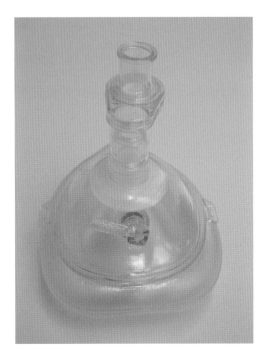

Figure 6.9 Pocket mask with an oxygen port.

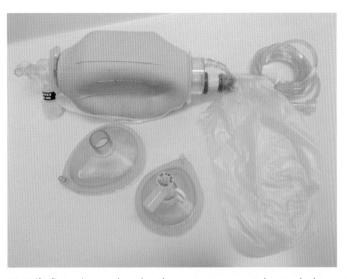

Figure 6.10 Self-inflating bag and mask with an oxygen reservoir bag and tubing with different size masks.

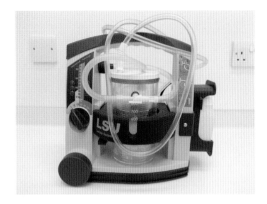

Figure 6.11 Portable suction.

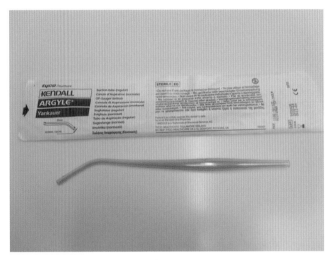

Figure 6.12 A Yankauer sucker.

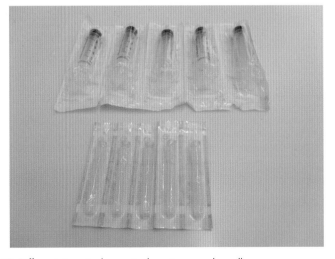

Figure 6.13 Different size, single-use sterile syringes and needles.

MEDICAL EMERGENCIES

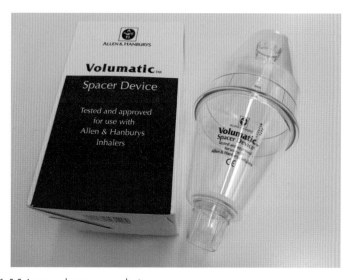

Figure 6.14 Large volume spacer device.

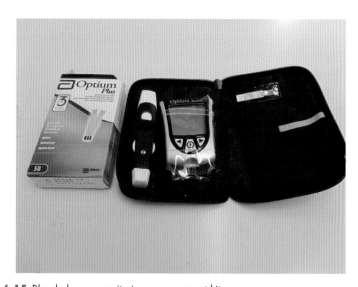

Figure 6.15 Blood glucose monitoring measurement kit.

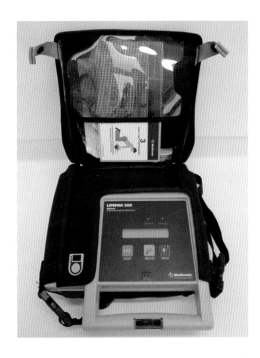

Figure 6.16 AED.

and the shock delivery time. A defibrillator should have recording facilities built in and standardised consumables such as self-adhesive pads and connecting cables [1].

COMMON MEDICAL EMERGENCIES

Common emergencies that can occur in the dental practice are as follows:

- Adrenal insufficiency
- Asthma
- Anaphylaxis
- Cardiac emergencies
- Choking and aspiration
- Epileptic seizures
- Hypoglycaemia
- Syncope (faint)

Asthma, angina, myocardial infarct, respiratory arrest, choking and aspiration can be categorised as conditions involving breathing difficulties and/or chest pain. Epilepsy and hypoglycaemia are conditions associated with fits. Anaphylaxis, adrenal insufficiency, faint and cardiac arrest are all conditions involving loss of consciousness [1].

MEDICAL EMERGENCIES

SIGNS AND SYMPTOMS OF MEDICAL EMERGENCIES

A sign is an indication that the patient is experiencing an emergency, as it would be observed, whereas a symptom is something the patient would experience enabling them, if it was a regular occurrence, to recognise that the condition was imminent.

MEDICAL EMERGENCIES

Adrenal insufficiency

Any patient who has been taking corticosteroids for any length of time, or has stopped taking them, can suffer adrenal insufficiency due to physiological stress, as this results in hypotension. As patients can become anxious at the thought of and actually receiving treatment there is a possibility that they may collapse because of this insufficiency. It is possible that routine dental treatment does not affect them so other reasons should not be ruled out when an assessment is made. A few patients have warning cards and by updating a patient's medical history it can be established whether they would require a prophylactic administration of steroids prior to treatment to prevent its occurrence [1,4,8].

Signs and symptoms of adrenal insufficiency
- Pale.
- A fall in blood pressure.
- A rapid loss of consciousness.
- Low blood glucose levels [1,4,8].

Management of adrenal insufficiency
- Patients should be laid flat with their legs higher than their head.
- Oxygen administered at 10–15L/min.
- Emergency services called.
- Monitored and reassured.
- Hydrocortisone administered [1,4,8].

Asthma attack

Asthma is a very common condition, which many sufferers make light of despite it affecting a large number of the population. However, it must be remembered that it can be life threatening. It is a chest condition which occurs due to narrowing of the airways where the lining of the walls swell and become inflamed. Occasionally sticky mucus and phlegm can attach to the airways making the tubes even narrower. Asthma attacks can occur because of stress, emotion, anxiety, exercise, being exposed to an allergen, colds or chest infections and laughter. Many people with asthma suffer from eczema and hay fever, with their condition being worsened during the hay fever season [1,5,8].

Signs and symptoms of an asthma attack
- Breathlessness.
- Inability to complete a sentence.
- Wheezing on exhalation.
- Accessory muscles of respiration in action.
- Increased respiratory rate (more than 25 per minute).
- Tachycardia, a fast pulse rate (more than 110 per minute).
- Anxiety [1,6].

Life threatening signs and symptoms
- Bradycardia, a slow pulse rate (less than 8 per minute).
- Decreased respiratory rate (less than 50 per minute).
- Cyanosis, blueness of the lips and/or extremities.
- Exhaustion, confusion and a decreased level of consciousness [1].

Management of an asthma attack
- Reassure the patient and sit them up. Do not lay the patient flat as this will increase their breathlessness.
- Patients normally carry their salbutamol (ventolin) inhaler (100mcg per activation) with them. They should be encouraged to take a few activations as this is usually all that is required. If they do not have their medication with them obtain it from the emergency drugs box. To eliminate the spread of infections the inhaler can be either given to the patient or discarded in the waste drugs box to be disposed of in the normal way.
- If a patient is unable to use their inhaler effectively, then additional doses should be given through a large volume spacer device.
- Call the emergency services if the patient does not improve or they exhibit life threatening signs and symptoms.
- If the patient's nebuliser is unavailable a large volume spacer device should be used with 4–6 activations of salbutamol being given and repeated every 10 minutes, as needed, until the emergency services arrive.
- While waiting for the emergency services maintain a patient's airway and administer oxygen at 10–15L/min.
- If a patient becomes unresponsive you should check for breathing and signs of life and if necessary undertake cardiopulmonary resuscitation, ignoring the occasional gasp.
- At all times patients must be monitored and reassured.

Any sick, cyanosed patient with respiratory difficulty should be administered a high flow of oxygen until the ambulance arrives as this is of benefit to them, even in the case of a patient who has chronic obstructive pulmonary disease. The benefit would outweigh any risks of causing respiratory depression [1].

Anaphylaxis

An anaphylactic shock is a type of hypersensitive reaction to otherwise unknown antigen (i.e. antibiotics, nuts). In dentistry, anaphylactic reactions may follow the administration of a drug or exposure to latex. It is caused by the release of histamine following an exposure to an antigen in a person who has previously been sensitised to that allergen. Anaphylactic reactions can also be attributed to additives and recipients in medicines, so it is vital to check the full contents of any which may contain fats and oils. Generally the more rapid the onset of the anaphylactic reaction the more serious the condition will be [1,8].

Signs and symptoms of anaphylaxis

Symptoms of an anaphylactic reaction can develop within minutes of exposure and early, effective management of this condition could be life saving. Unfortunately, as there are a huge range of possible signs and symptoms it can make the condition very difficult to diagnose:

- Urticaria (an itchy skin eruption which is characterised by weals that have pale interiors with well-defined red margins).
- Rhinitis (an inflammation of the mucous membrane lining the nose).
- Conjunctivitis (inflammation of the conjunctiva of the eye).
- Nausea, vomiting, diarrhoea and abdominal pains.
- Patients experience a sense of unease and impending doom.
- Flushing is very common – however a pale complexion may also occur.
- Marked upper airway (laryngeal).
- Oedema (swelling) of the tongue and upper airway.
- Bronchospasms may develop, causing strider (a whistling noise on inspiration and wheezing).
- Peripheral coldness and cold clammy skin.
- Rapid/weak impalpable pulse, tachycardia with a rapid drop in blood pressure.
- Vasodilation leading to a drop in the blood pressure and collapse.
- Respiratory arrest (breathing has stopped, but circulation is still present).
- Loss of consciousness and cardiac arrest [1,8].

Management of anaphylaxis

First-line treatment

- Remove the item that has caused the reaction and if a drug was being administered stop its use immediately.

- Immediately place the patient in the supine position to restore their blood pressure.
- Maintain the patient's airway and administer oxygen at 10–15L/min [1,8].

Severe reaction

- Call the emergency services.
- A semi-conscious patient or one presenting severe bronchospasms and a widespread rash should have a 0.5ml adrenaline injection 1:1000 administered intramuscularly (IM) in either their outer arm or thigh.
- An auto-injector (epipen) preparation of adrenaline is available as a 0.3ml injection, 1:1000 for self-administration by a patient who is aware that they will have a severe reaction. If the patient has his/her epipen and it is immediately available then it is acceptable to use it.
- The dose of adrenaline should be repeated every 5 minutes according to the patient's blood pressure, respiratory and pulse rates.
- At all times monitor and reassure the patient.
- If the patient loses consciousness they should be assessed for signs of life and breathing and, if necessary, undertake cardiopulmonary resuscitation, ignoring the occasional gasp.
- All patients should be transferred to hospital for further assessment, irrespective of their initial recovery.
- An antihistamine drug, chlorpheniramine maleate (Piriton) and steroid, hydrocortisone succinate (Solu-cortef) are useful in the management of an allergic reaction but they are not first-line drugs and will be administered by the emergency services if necessary [1,8].

Children

The dose of intramuscular adrenaline 1:1000 is based on the approximate age of the child or their weight:

- 12 years – 500mcg IM (0.5ml)
- If child is small or pre-pubertal – 250mcg
- 6–12 years – 250mcg IM (0.25ml)
- 6 months to 6 years – 120mcg IM (0.12ml)
- 6 months –50mcg (0.05ml)

Less severe cases and asthma sufferers

- Any patient wheezing or experiencing difficulty breathing can be treated with a few activations of a salbutamol inhaler and if necessary a large volume spacer device can be used with 4–6 activations of salbutamol being administered. This can be repeated every 10 minutes until the emergency services arrive.

MEDICAL EMERGENCIES

- If the patient shows signs and symptoms that are life threatening then intramuscular adrenaline can be administered [1].

CARDIAC EMERGENCIES

Cardiac emergencies cover a range of conditions. These are:

- Angina pectoris
- Myocardial infarct
- Cardiac arrest

All chest pain should be treated seriously even if it is suspected that the patient is suffering from indigestion, because indigestion can be extremely painful and distressing for the patient and can quite easily be mistaken for a cardiac emergency. Normally acute chest pain is caused by an angina attack or a myocardial infarction [1,8].

Signs and symptoms of acute chest pain

- Severe crushing chest pain.
- Vomiting.
- Breathlessness.
- An increased respiratory rate.
- Pulse may be weak (irregular or regular).
- Low blood pressure and an altered mental state.
- Loss of consciousness [1,8].

Management of acute chest pain

- Do not lay these patients flat as this increases their breathlessness.
- Reassure and monitor the patient.
- If the patient is a known angina sufferer then they should be carrying their medication, glyceryl trinitrate spray with them. Encourage and help them to use it. If they do not have their medication with them obtain it from the emergency drugs box. To eliminate the spread of infections the glyceryl trinitrate spray can be either given to the patient or discarded in the waste drugs box to be disposed of in the normal way.
- Administer oxygen if necessary at 10–15L/min, adjusting the flow rate as required according to the patient's response.
- Monitor the patient's vital signs for any sign of regression, as the diagnosis would then need to be reconsidered and treated accordingly.
- If required a 300mg aspirin can be administered orally – either crushed or chewed. If an aspirin is administered then the emergency services should be made aware of this.

- If the patient becomes unresponsive, assess breathing and check for signs of life and, if necessary, undertake cardiopulmonary resuscitation, ignoring the occasional gasp.
- In the event that an attack is severe and/or the patient is distressed, then call for an ambulance [1,8].

Angina attack

Angina occurs when heart muscles do not receive enough oxygen-rich blood, which results in chest pain or discomfort which can be likened to indigestion. Angina is not a disease but an indication of an underlying heart problem with the most common being coronary artery disease. It can be caused by myocardial ischaemia, exercise, stress and hypertension [1,2,8].

Signs and symptoms of an angina attack
- Severe retrosternal pain, possibly radiating down the left arm and into the neck. Pain can also be experienced in the right arm.
- Pain or tightness in the centre of the chest.
- Pulse can be regular or irregular.
- Shortness of breath.
- Sweating.
- Nausea.
- Light-headedness.
- Feeling weak.
- Women are more prone to experiencing pain in their back, shoulders and abdomen [1,8].

Management of an angina attack
- Reassure patient and sit them up. Laying a patient down would increase their breathlessness and pain.
- Encourage the patient to use their glyceryl trinitrate spray sublingually. If necessary the clinician can administer it.
- Maintain the patient's airway and administer oxygen at 10–15L/min.
- Glyceryl trinitrate can be repeated three times.
- If there is no relief for the patient after 3 minutes consider a myocardial infarction and administer a 300mg aspirin.
- Call the emergency services [1,2,8].

Myocardial infarction

When blood flow is blocked to any part of the heart muscle a heart attack may be imminent and if that flow of blood is not restored quickly part of the heart muscle becomes damaged and begins to die due to lack of oxygen. Coronary artery disease occurs when the insides of the arteries become coated with a

MEDICAL EMERGENCIES

fatty material known as plaque, which on rupturing can lead to a blood clot forming. If this clot increases in size it can cause narrowing or a complete blockage in the blood pathway to the heart muscle, limiting the oxygen-rich blood, thereby causing myocardial infarction which is commonly known as a heart attack [1,6,8].

Signs and symptoms of a myocardial infarction
- Severe crushing retrosternal chest pain down the left arm radiating up into the neck. Pain can be experienced in the right arm.
- Breathlessness.
- Nausea and vomiting.
- Pale and clammy skin and extreme distress.
- Weak, irregular pulse and low blood pressure.
- Deathly appearance.
- Loss of consciousness.
- Cardiac arrest [1,6,8].

Management of a myocardial infarction
- Call the emergency services.
- Reassurance is very important in order that the patient remains as calm as possible.
- Place the patient in the most comfortable position, which is usually sitting up. If the patient feels faint, then lay them flat and restore their blood pressure by raising their legs slightly above their heart.
- Maintain their airway and administer oxygen at the rate of 10–15L/min through a Hudson mask.
- Some clinicians may decide to administer 50% oxygen and 50% nitrous oxide via a relative analgesia machine, because on mixing they form the gas entonox. The nitrous oxide will provide a patient with some pain relief because of its mild analgesic properties. It will also provide some amnesia – therefore the patient will not remember some of the pain experienced during the attack.
- Administer a 300mg aspirin to thin the blood.
- If necessary assist the patient in the administration of a glyceryl trinitrate spray.
- Continually monitor the patient and watch for signs of a cardiac arrest, performing cardiopulmonary resuscitation if the patient loses consciousness, stops breathing and/or doesn't show any signs of life [1,6,8].

Cardiac arrest

If the patient's heart suddenly stops functioning a cardiac arrest would occur and death would follow within minutes of the signs and symptoms appearing. A patient who suffers a cardiac arrest may or may not have previously been diagnosed with having a heart condition. However, the most common under-lying factor for a patient to die suddenly from cardiac arrest is coronary heart disease. Many cardiac arrests that cause sudden death occur as a result of the electrical impulses in the diseased heart becoming rapid (ventricular tachycar-dia), chaotic (ventricular fibrillation) or sometimes even both and as a result the irregular heart rhythm (arrhythmia) causes the heart to suddenly stop beat-ing. Some cardiac arrests can be attributed to the heart rate slowing down, known as bradycardia. Other reasons for cardiac arrest are respiratory arrest, drowning, electrocution, choking, hypoxia, trauma and it can occur without any contributing factors. A cardiac arrest can be reversible provided the patient experiencing it is treated immediately and certainly within a few minutes by an electric shock to the heart to restore the heartbeat to normal. This is known as defibrillation and will increase the patient's chance of survival. A patient will start to suffer brain death and permanent death within 4–6 minutes of experiencing a cardiac arrest and sadly very few attempts at resuscitating a patient after 10 minutes are successful [1,7,8].

Signs and symptoms of a cardiac arrest
- No signs of life.
- No breathing/abnormal breathing in the form of infrequent noisy gasps.
- Unconsciousness [1,7,8].

Management of a cardiac arrest for an adult
- Check the surrounding area for any danger/hazards that might harm you, because if you are injured it could be difficult to help the patient.
- Assess the responsiveness of the patient by touching both their shoulders and speaking into both ears with authority, asking them if they are okay, but do not shout.
- Call for help from anyone in the vicinity. If someone appears ask them to fetch an AED, if one is available. When an AED is used interruptions to chest compressions should be kept to a minimum.
- Open the patient's airway by tilting their head and lifting their chin.
- Check for any debris that may be in the patient's mouth and if it is easily accessible remove it, being careful not to push it backwards into their oropharynx and possibly further into the airway which could cause a blockage. Suction may be required to remove any secretions. If the patient is wearing dentures and they are a good fit, leave them in. This helps to main-tain the shape of the patient's mouth and face, but remove any ill-fitting ones.
- Assess the patient's breathing by observation and by placing your cheek close to theirs, feeling for any breath on your cheek to establish if there is any chest movement. At the same time look for any signs of life and ignore any occasional gasps or abnormal breathing.

MEDICAL EMERGENCIES

- At this stage the emergency services should be called. If you are still alone, because nobody has responded to your call for help you will have to leave the patient to contact them. If somebody has arrived to help, one of you should make the call and return to advise that the emergency services are on their way, while the other commences cardiopulmonary resuscitation.
- If on your own: Upon returning to the patient 30 chest compressions should be performed at a depth of 5–6cm (third of the chest) over the sternum and at a rate of 100–120 per minute followed by two ventilations.
- Do not stop cardiopulmonary resuscitation until the emergency services arrive unless the patient shows signs of regaining consciousness, they move and start to breathe normally, open their eyes or cough [1,7,8].

Management of a cardiac arrest for a child
- Assess the patient in the same way as you would an adult.
- If the child is not breathing normally then administer five rescue breaths.
- If the child is still unresponsive and doesn't exhibit any sign of life/circulation, then, before calling the emergency services you should carry out 1 minute of cardiopulmonary resuscitation by performing 15 chest compressions and two rescue breaths, using one or two hands for a child over the age of 1 to achieve an adequate depth of at least one third of the chest [1,8].

Management of a cardiac arrest due to electrocution, drowning, trauma or other causes
The patient is treated in the same way as a child, adjusting the ratio of compressions to ventilations to suit the age of the patient [1,8].

Additional information
The aim of providing basic life support to a patient who is in cardiac arrest is to sustain life until the advanced life support/emergency services arrive.

Chest compressions
- Artificially circulates the oxygen around the body.
- The pressure provided should be firm, controlled and applied vertically. Erratic or violent compressions are dangerous.
- Time should not be wasted feeling for the carotid pulse as the chances of recovery are slim without advanced life support. However, if the patient moves or takes a spontaneous breath, then check for any sign of life [7,8].

Ventilations
- Each inflation should take approximately 1–2 seconds with only a small amount of resistance being felt. If you inflate too quickly less air will go into the lungs.

- The tidal volume aimed for is approximately 800–1200ml in an adult.
- The chest must fall before inflation is given. This normally takes around 1–2 seconds [7, 8].

If a patient is not breathing but shows signs of life

If it is established that a collapsed patient is exhibiting signs of life but not breathing, they are experiencing a condition known as **respiratory arrest** [1]. To manage this condition you should do the following:

- Call the emergency services.
- Administer 10–12 effective breaths and recheck for signs of life to make certain they are present.
- If breathing is restored, place the patient in the recovery position and monitor for any sign of deterioration. In the event of the patient's breathing disappearing you should place him/her onto their back and resume rescue breathing.
- If the patient's signs of life disappear, you should commence cardiopulmonary resuscitation as previously explained [1,7,8].

CHOKING AND ASPIRATION

In dentistry the oropharynx is susceptible to items falling into it, especially if it is not protected by the use of rubber dam and high volume aspiration during procedures using small items [1].

Signs and symptoms of choking and aspiration

- Coughing and spluttering.
- Breathing difficulties.
- Noisy breathing (wheezing and strider).
- Paradoxical chest (where during breathing all or part of the lungs inflate during inhalation and balloons out during exhalation) or abdominal movements.
- Cyanosis.
- Loss of consciousness [1].

Management of aspiration

- Sit the patient up and reassure them.
- Encourage them to cough.
- Ask them to search their clothing to see if the item has fallen on it or within it.

MEDICAL EMERGENCIES

- Look on the floor to see if it has fallen.
- If the practice has the facility to X-ray the suction tubing and pot, then this can be undertaken to eliminate the possibility that it was aspirated into the suction equipment.
- If the item cannot be found then the patient should be sent as an emergency for a chest X-ray, to establish whether it has ended up in the stomach or the lungs. If it were to fall into the lungs it would be more likely to go into the right lung due to the anatomy of the respiratory tract. This is because the right bronchus is straighter than the left and higher up, due to the diaphragm being slightly higher on the right than on the left.
- If the patient is wheezing a few activations of a salbutamol inhaler may help [1].

Management of choking

- If the blockage is partial then the patient will usually, through coughing, be able to dislodge it. However, if there is a complete blockage then this may not be possible.
- If a patient has a partial blockage, he/she will be distressed and coughing with a respiratory wheeze.
- If a patient has a full blockage, he/she will be unable to speak, breathe or cough, which will eventually lead to a loss of consciousness.
- If the patient is breathing then he/she should be encouraged to cough.
- If the patient exhibits any signs of becoming weak, stops coughing or breathing then they are to be left in the position they are in.
- If possible remove any obvious foreign objects carefully.
- Whether the patient is standing or sitting you should stand to the side of them, but slightly behind and support with one hand. Lean him/her forward and administer five sharp slaps between the shoulder blades, using the base of the palm of your hand. These slaps should be fairly forceful and in an upward action. As soon as the object is expelled from the patient's mouth you must stop the back slaps.
- If the back slaps fail to remove the object then five abdominal thrusts are recommended to be undertaken, as follows:
  - Whether the patient is standing or sitting, position yourself behind him/her and place both your arms around the upper part of their abdomen, clench your fist and place it between the umbilicus (belly button) and xiphisternum (lower part of the sternum), grasp it with your other hand and pull it sharply inwards and upwards five times. If the object is expelled from the patient's mouth you must stop the abdominal thrusts.
  - If the patient is lying down, kneel beside them and roll them onto their side, then onto your legs. Support their chest and protect their head by holding their chin and apply five back slaps, as previously explained. If

MEDICAL EMERGENCIES

the object is not expelled, then turn them so that they are once again flat on their backs and kneel astride them, placing your hands in the position previously explained and thrust sharply downwards towards the patient's head.

- If the patient becomes unconscious, then call the emergency services and carry out cardiopulmonary resuscitation, adjusting the sequence to suit the age of the patient [1,8].

EPILEPSY

Anyone can suffer from epilepsy and it can start at any age. It is the most common serious neurological condition affecting people in the United Kingdom and worldwide. It is different from other neurological conditions as the seizures tend to start from the brain. Stress, tiredness, bright lights, starvation, menstruation, some drugs and alcohol are some of the triggers that can affect certain individuals, causing them to have an epileptic seizure even though they are well controlled by their medication. Most fits terminate spontaneously [1,3,8].

Signs and symptoms of epilepsy

- The patient may have a brief warning or an aura (sensation).
- The patient can look and feel detached from their surroundings.
- The patient will suddenly lose consciousness.
- The patient will become rigid, fall to the ground and may cry out and in the tonic phase they can become cyanosed. After a few seconds, his/her limbs jerk in thrashing movements and the tongue may be bitten in the clonic phase.
- There may be frothing at the mouth and the patient may become urinary incontinent.
- The seizure will last for a few minutes and once over the patient may become very floppy and remain unconscious.
- Recovery will be very slow and can be variable, with some individuals left feeling very dazed and confused. Most patients will try to get up as soon as they recover but they must be allowed time to rest before being discharged into the care of a responsible adult [1,3,8].

It must be remembered that a fit can be associated with hypoglycaemia and fainting. Therefore, by the use of a blood glucose measurement kit and by taking and recording a pulse and blood pressure these medical conditions can be ruled out [1].

MEDICAL EMERGENCIES

Management of epilepsy

- Prevent the patient from injuring themselves by removing all equipment, materials and medicaments from the immediate area.
- The patient's head can be placed on a pillow or you can place your hands either side of their head to cushion it as it moves from side to side.
- Do not place anything between the patient's teeth or insert an airway whilst they are having convulsions.
- Maintain the patient's airway and administer oxygen at 10–15L/min.
- Do not, at any time, try to restrain the patient as this could cause an unnecessary injury.
- When the patient recovers, place him/her in the recovery position and monitor their vital signs.
- Patients may be confused and will, therefore, require verbal reassurance.
- Patients should not be discharged until they are fully recovered.
- If the patient remains unconscious, check for breathing (ignoring the occasional gasp) and signs of life and if necessary and commence cardiopulmonary resuscitation.
- If the patient does not recover after 5 minutes or the convulsive movements recur in quick succession, then the emergency services should be called, because the patient could have status epilepticus.
- The emergency services can administer 10mg of diazepam IM to a patient over 10 years, 7.5mg to a child aged 5–10 years and 5mg to a child aged 1–5 years (immediately through the patient's clothes, either into the thigh or the upper arm). An alternative drug that can be administered into the buccal sulcus is Epistatus (midazolam) (Figure 6.17). It is available as 10mg/ml [1,3,8].

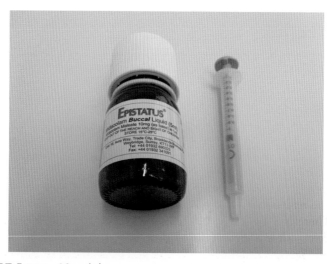

Figure 6.17 Epistatus 10mg/ml.

MEDICAL EMERGENCIES

HYPOGLYCAEMIA

A hypoglycaemic episode can be caused by poorly controlled diabetes mellitus, a missed meal, an infection or fever. Patients who suffer from diabetes should eat normally, taking their normal dose of insulin or oral hypoglycaemic agent before attending for any scheduled treatment. If a patient does not have food after insulin, their blood glucose will fall to a low level (hypoglycaemia). However, some patients may exhibit symptoms at higher blood sugar levels. Patients usually recognise the signs and symptoms and will manage hypoglycaemia themselves. However, children may not recognise the signs and symptoms and they may not be as obvious as in an adult. One feature they may exhibit is lethargy [1,8].

Signs and symptoms of hypoglycaemia

- Irritability and aggressiveness.
- Uncooperative, truculent and have slurred speech.
- Cold, clammy, sweaty skin, complaint of a headache and possibly shaking and trembling.
- Drowsiness, disorientation, difficulty in concentrating, be vague and confused.
- Fitting and gradual loss of consciousness [1,8].

Management of hypoglycaemia

To confirm that a patient is experiencing a hypoglycaemic episode, their blood glucose level should be taken and depending upon the outcome, the status of the patient and their vital signs, it may be necessary to call the emergency services immediately [1,8].

The early stage

If the patient is cooperative and conscious they can be provided with either a glucose drink, milk with some added sugar, dextrose tablets or gel, repeating this after 10–15 minutes if necessary.

The severe stage

If the patient's level of consciousness is impaired, they become uncooperative or are unable to swallow, then either buccal glucose gel and/or glucagon IM should be administered by the clinician as follows:

- 1mg to adults and 0.5mg to children under 8 years.
- The blood glucose level needs to be retaken after 10 minutes using a blood glucose monitoring kit to ensure it has risen. The patient should be monitored to ensure their level of consciousness has improved.
- Once the patient is responsive, coercive and feels able to swallow then either oral glucose or some form of high-carbohydrate food should be provided.

MEDICAL EMERGENCIES

- When the patient has recovered he/she may be discharged into the care of a responsible escort and must be advised not to drive themselves.
- Transfer the patient to hospital, if necessary.
- If a patient becomes unresponsive at any time, check for signs of life and undertake cardiopulmonary resuscitation, ignoring any occasional gasps. If not already done call the emergency services before commencing.
- It can take 5–10 minutes for glucagon to take effect, as it requires adequate glucose stores within the body for it to be effective. Consequently, it may be ineffective with anorexic and alcoholic patients [1,8].

FAINTING/SYNCOPE

Fainting is the most common cause of sudden and temporary loss of consciousness in the surgery. It is also known as a vasovagal attack or syncope. It is either caused by hypotension or inadequate cerebral perfusion to the brain, therefore less oxygen, any of which results in the patient losing consciousness. Factors that can cause patients to faint include anxiety, pain, fatigue, fasting, high temperature, relative humidity and during or after administration of a local anaesthetic. It must be remembered that although some patients are prone to fainting and that it is a common cause of collapse, that upon recovery a patient may feel stressed at its occurrence. Patients can faint due to other reasons, such as standing for long periods of time or rising too quickly. Patients who are taking prescribed medication for hypertension are more at risk of fainting and should be allowed to take their time when getting out of the dental chair. When a patient is stressed and anxious they may hyperventilate, where they will experience light-headedness or faintness. This does not normally lead to fainting, but can progress to tetany (muscle spasms in the face and hands) if not managed. In this situation all that is normally required is good patient management and reassurance [1,8].

Signs and symptoms of a faint/syncope

- Pallor (putty colour).
- Dizziness.
- Light headed and feeling weak.
- Blurred vision.
- Nausea and vomiting.
- Sweating, especially on the brow and upper lip.
- Complaining of being hot, thirsty and yawning.
- Pulse will initially be slow and weak, then rapid due to the blood pressure being low.
- Loss of consciousness and a limp patient [1,8].

Management of a faint/syncope

- Lower the patient's head by laying him/her down with legs raised to improve the venous return. This increases the blood flow to the brain. If the patient is pregnant or obese, then lay them on their left side to avoid squashing the vena cava's of the heart and to avoid restricting their breathing.
- Loosen clothing, especially around the neck and administer oxygen at 10–15L/min, explaining your actions at all times.
- Apply a cold compress to the head and increase ventilation in the surgery.
- Upon recovery, provide the patient with a glucose drink.
- Discuss deferring treatment.
- At all times monitor and reassure the patient and talk to him/her as the hearing is the last sense to be lost and the first one to return.
- If the patient does not recover within 2–3 minutes re-diagnose the situation and if necessary, call the emergency services – in the absence of breathing, ignoring the occasional gasp and signs of life, prepare to undertake cardiopulmonary resuscitation.

NOTE

The dental nurse is reminded that they must not under any circumstances draw up or administer drugs. The only situation in which a drug may be drawn up by a dental nurse is during a medical emergency and even then it must only be under the supervision of the clinician.

AIRWAY CONTROL AND VENTILATION

During an emergency the nurse should, if required, assist the clinician with the preparation and insertion of airway adjuncts so that the patient receives adequate oxygenation at all times to ensure that their brain and vital organs are not damaged. An airway adjunct will maintain an open airway for a patient who has lost consciousness. It is vital that once a diagnosis has been established by assessing for signs of life and breathing and it has been recognised that an airway adjunct would be life saving, one should be inserted. It must be remembered that basic airway management – by tilting the patient's head, chin lift and jaw thrust – should be undertaken first, as this may be all that is required, coupled with the use of suction. Once an airway is inserted there are various masks that can be used to oxygenate patients [8].

Airways used

- Oropharyngeal airways (Figure 6.8)
- Nasopharyngeal airways (Figure 6.18) [8]

MEDICAL EMERGENCIES

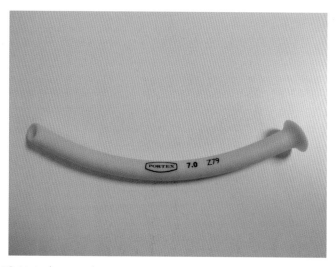

Figure 6.18 Nasopharyngeal airway.

Equipment used

- Pocket mask
- Self-inflating bag mask valve
- Oxygen [8]

Other equipment used

- Hudson mask (Figure 6.19)
- Nasal cannula (Figure 6.20) [8]

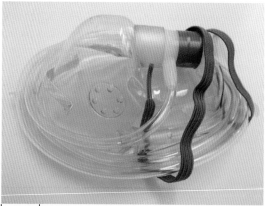

Figure 6.19 Hudson mask.

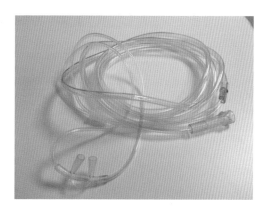

Figure 6.20 Nasal cannula.

Possible causes of an airway obstruction

Airway obstructions can occur at any time and, as previously explained, can be either partial or complete. In an unconscious patient the most common area that can be obstructed is the pharynx, which can quite easily be occluded by the tongue. However, it should be remembered that other factors can also be responsible for airway obstructions such as the epiglottis, soft palate, vomit and oedema. Trauma or inhalation of a foreign body can lead to blood in that area, possibly leading to a laryngeal obstruction. Airway obstruction below the larynx is not as common – however, it can occur for reasons such as aspiration of the gastric contents or the patient experiencing bronchospasms [8].

Signs and symptoms of an airway obstruction

As with any emergency, the patient has to be assessed by the conventional 'look at the chest and abdominal areas to establish if there is any movement, **listen** to and **feel** for any airflow coming from the mouth and nose' method as well as by looking/checking for any signs of life. When a partial obstruction is experienced the air movement is reduced and invariably noisy. An upper airway obstruction will cause inspiratory stridor, with any expiratory noise suggesting that there is an obstruction to the lower airway as it is prone to collapse and obstructing during expiration. A patient might snore if the pharynx is partially blocked by the tongue, whereas a crowing noise will be heard during a laryngeal spasm and if a liquid or a semi-solid foreign body is present then a gurgling noise would be heard. A patient who has a complete blockage who is attempting to breathe will exhibit paradoxical chest and abdominal movements, which can often be enhanced by the use of their accessory respiratory muscles. As this action can look normal, it is important to look for/establish the absence of breathing before diagnosing this condition [8].

How to clear a blocked airway

As soon as it has been established that the patient has an obstruction, whether it be partial or complete, action should be immediately taken to open and maintain a clear airway. This is undertaken by using the simple technique of tilting the head and lifting the chin, or if necessary a jaw thrust [8].

Head tilt and chin lift

By lifting a patient's head the neck, muscles lift the base of the tongue from the posterior pharyngeal wall and the epiglottis away from the laryngeal inlet. By lifting their chin (Figure 6.21) it stretches them even further, pulling the mandible and therefore the tongue forward. To undertake this technique the patient's head needs to be extended by pushing the forehead backwards and the occiput caudally, while at the same time placing two fingers under the tip of the patient's mandible to lift their chin, displacing their tongue anteriorly. If it is suspected that the patient has suffered a neck injury, the head can be tilted only if other methods of opening the airway have been unsuccessful. It is important to bear in mind that neck movements should be limited to avoid worsening the injury and that death, through hypoxia, is more likely to occur than tetraplegia as a result of maintaining a patient's airway during an emergency. In this instance a jaw thrust can be used [8].

Jaw thrust

A jaw thrust (Figure 6.22) is an alternative procedure for relieving an obstruction caused by the tongue. It can also be used if it is thought that the patient has

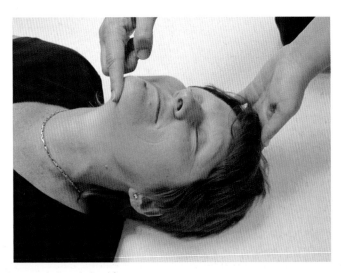

Figure 6.21 Head tilt and chin lift position.

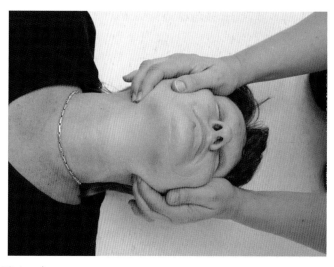

Figure 6.22 Jaw thrust.

a nasal obstruction, as the mouth would then provide an airway. To undertake this technique the patient's mouth must be slightly open. The thumbs need to be placed on the chin so that it can be displaced downwards. At the same time the fingers are positioned behind the angle of the mandible. Pressure should be applied in an upward and forward action so that the jaw is lifted forwards. The head tilt, chin lift and the jaw thrust are successful in almost all cases when the airway obstruction is a result of the soft tissues relaxing. Whichever technique is used it is important to ensure that the airway is patent by the looking, listening and feeling process, because if it is not, then other possible causes should be explored and managed [8].

Airways

Airways are adjuncts that are often helpful and can be vital in maintaining a patient's airway, especially when or if resuscitation is expected to be prolonged. Oropharyngeal and nasopharyngeal airways are tubes that are manufactured to ensure that when placed in situ the patient's tongue is not displaced backwards and the airway is kept open. The head tilt, chin lift or jaw thrust is required in conjunction with an airway adjunct so that they continue to be aligned and functional. The action of opening a patient's airway by the method previously explained, or after insertion of either of the airway adjuncts, the patient's breathing should be restored spontaneously. They should then be placed in the recovery position. By placing a patient in this position, it not only puts them in a stable position but also reduces any risk of further blockages and permits any secretions, such as vomit or blood to drain away from the upper airway.

MEDICAL EMERGENCIES

It is imperative that oxygen is administered and that the patient is continually reassured and monitored for any signs of regression [8].

Oropharyngeal airways

These airways are curved plastic tubes which are flanged and reinforced at the oral end. They are flat in shape and consequently fit comfortably between the tongue and the hard palate. Various sizes are available, suitable for newborn babies up to large adults. To estimate the size to be inserted the chosen airway is measured by placing one end on the angle of the patient's mandible with the other at the corner of the patient's mouth [8].

Insertion of an oropharyngeal airway

Insertion into a patient's airway is undertaken only by clinicians and they will only attempt to place one if the patient is comatosed. The reason for this is: If the patient's glossopharyngeal and laryngeal reflexes are functioning the patient may vomit or experience a laryngeal spasm and the tongue may be forced backwards exacerbating the obstruction. Before an airway is inserted it must be established that there are no foreign bodies in the patient's mouth that could be forced into the larynx. If necessary suction equipment could be used to remove any secretions. The airway is held in the inverted position and placed into the oral cavity, rotated 180° as it passes below the palate and into the oropharynx. If an airway is placed incorrectly the tongue could be pushed further backwards and possibly into the pharynx causing the airway to be obstructed. If at any time the patient retches or coughs the airway should be removed to prevent a laryngeal spasm or vomiting. Once it is inserted the head and neck must be correctly positioned using the head tilt, chin lift or jaw thrust method, ensuring that the look, listen and feel procedure is undertaken and that the patency of the airway is providing adequate ventilation [8].

Nasopharyngeal airways

These airways are life saving in patients who have trismus, clenched jaws, suffered trauma, have a possible maxillary fracture or have limited mouth opening, because the placement of this type of airway does not involve insertion into the mouth, but into the nasal passage. It is thought that they are better tolerated than oropharyngeal airways. However, they should not be used on a patient who exhibits signs and symptoms of a fractured base of the skull. They are made of malleable plastic which is bevelled at one end with a flange at the other and as the internal diameter of the airway increases so does the length of the tube. To select the size required for a patient the bevelled end is measured against the patient's little finger to establish whether the internal diameter of the airway is approximately the same size. On insertion it can cause the patient's nose to bleed and if the airway is too long the patient could vomit or experience a laryngeal spasm [8].

Insertion of a nasopharyngeal airway

Once again, insertion is undertaken only by clinicians. The patency of the right nostril must firstly be checked to ensure it is not blocked. If it is then the left nostril can be checked and used instead. A safety pin depending upon the size of the flange may have to be fixed into that area to prevent the airway being inhaled. The airway is then inserted, bevelled end into the right nostril using a rotating action to twist it into the airway along the floor of the nose. When fully inserted the bevelled end should sit in the pharynx with the flange resting at the nostril. If at any time an obstruction is felt or any difficulty in insertion is encountered then it should be removed and the left nostril should be used. Once it is inserted the head and neck must be correctly positioned using the head tilt, chin lift or jaw thrust method, ensuring that the look, listen and feel procedure is undertaken to ensure the patency of the airway [8].

Means of administering oxygen

Ideally, artificial ventilation should be commenced immediately for any patient when spontaneous ventilation is found to be inadequate or absent by carrying out mouth-to-mouth resuscitation without the use of any resuscitation equipment. However, some people may find the thought of direct mouth-to-mouth contact with another person unpleasant, especially if there is blood or vomit present around the mouth area. Mouth-to-mouth resuscitation is not recommended – therefore various types of equipment are available to assist with providing patients with ventilatory support.

Oxygen information

Oxygen is a clear, colourless and odourless medical gas which is administered to patients under the direction of a clinician during an emergency in order to support life. It is not categorised as being flammable but it will support combustion. Care must be taken when storing and handling cylinders. It is supplied in cylinders that are painted black with a white collar, at a pressure of approximately 2000psi. It is supplied in various-size cylinders – C, D, E, F and G. If a patient attends for treatment and they are on oxygen therapy they should be transferred as soon as possible to piped oxygen (if available). Patients must receive an adequate amount of oxygen, as it is essential to sustain life. When storing cylinders the full and empty ones must be separated, with the full stock being kept in date order to avoid expiry going unnoticed. During transportation a trolley should be used to avoid injuries. Never smoke when oxygen cylinders are present and avoid using hand cream, because when oxygen is under high pressure and grease or oil is present there is a possibility of explosion/combustion. Never attempt to lubricate any of the connections, valves or fitments. On all cylinders a plastic collar is fitted which informs the user of the size of the cylinder, batch number, expiry date and contents, so there can be no doubt what they contain. Always look for confirmation to avoid the wrong gas being administered. The flow meter must be cared for to ensure that it is not leaking. It must always be kept vertical, ensuring that the ball contained within lifts and rotates. It should never be dismantled for cleaning, but just wiped over with a cloth and it must always be switched off when not in use. With piped oxygen the hose should be changed every 3–5 years as they can become worn. They must never be repaired in-house by the use of tape. The vulnerable part of the hose is the neck, which could combust. When not in use it should be removed with care by holding it to avoid ejection at high speed. It must be stored properly to avoid accidents. When reconnecting the hose it must be checked to ensure that it is not crushed or tangled, as this will reduce the flow of oxygen that a patient receives [8].

Laerdal pocket mask
A Laerdal pocket mask is used during mouth-to-mouth resuscitation to administer oxygen to a patient who has collapsed. It avoids the need of direct patient-to-user contact by providing a barrier, thereby minimising cross infection. These are see through masks, which enable the user to see any condensation in the event of a patient's respiration being restored. They have 'nose' imprinted on them to avoid them being applied to the patient's face the incorrect way. They also have a spongy base which allows flexibility and achieves a good seal, a disposable one-way valve which prevents the back flow of any of the patient's expired air to the user and an oxygen port with which to attach tubing. This can be used to increase the oxygen percentage a patient receives. If the Laerdal pocket mask is used without oxygen attached, a patient will receive the user's expired oxygen, which is 16%, but with supplementary oxygen being provided at a flow rate of 6–7L/min the oxygen received by the patient will be increased to 65–70%. The maximum flow rate an oxygen cylinder can deliver is 15L/min. However, when using a Laerdal pocket mask with the oxygen turned to maximum the oxygen tubing could possibly become detached from the cylinder. This would mean that the patient would receive interrupted oxygen. It is therefore preferable to have a continuous flow at a reduced rate. Some older masks do not have an oxygen port so the oxygen tube can be placed directly under the mask to provide additional oxygen to a patient. Disposable masks are also available [8].

Hudson mask
A Hudson mask is used to administer supplementary oxygen to a patient during the recovery stage of either a collapsed patient or after a patient has received a general anaesthetic. They are disposable and are available in various sizes. They are made of clear plastic and have exhalation holes with some having reservoir bags. There is a metal strip over the nose area and an elastic strap which allows the mask to sit comfortably over the patient's nose and mouth

area without the need for it to be held in place. The flow rate will depend upon the clinical diagnosis and condition of the patient, but would be set at approximately 3–6L/min [8].

Bag mask valve

Formerly known as an ambu bag. When using a bag mask valve it is more effective for two people rather than one to use it as it is very technique sensitive. It must only be used by staff members that have been trained in its use. They are ideal when a patient suffers cardiac arrest, being no need for the user to inhale into the mask. The action of squeezing the valve provides the pressure to inflate the lungs. They are supplied with different size valves and some are disposable. Different size masks are also available. They have a port to attach an oxygen supply and when they are not connected to a cylinder they will provide a patient with 21% oxygen which is the air concentration. This percentage can be increased by connecting the port to an oxygen cylinder, turning the flow rate up to 15L/min and attaching a reservoir bag to the mask and valve which will increase the percentage a patient receives to approximately 80–85%, because the oxygen is stored within the bag. However, if a reservoir bag is not available the percentage of oxygen a patient will receive is approximately 50% [8].

Nasal cannula

A nasal cannula is a clear plastic tube which has two prongs that are designed to be placed within a patient's nose, allowing supplementary oxygen to be provided during treatment with the mouth area free for access. Patients who are on long-term oxygen therapy will also use this adjunct to receive supplementary oxygen which is vital. The flow rate is normally set at approximately 4–5L/min, but patients who are transferred from the oxygen cylinder that they normally use to a piped system will advise if the amount of oxygen they are receiving is too little or too much [8].

CONCLUSION

If a patient collapsed and you were on your own the preferred adjunct would be to use a Laerdal pocket mask attached to an oxygen cylinder with a flow rate of 6–7L/min. This provides a patient with 65–70% oxygen. However, if you have undergone the appropriate training and are at the competency level to use a bag mask valve attached to an oxygen cylinder at a flow rate of 15L/min, the percentage would increase to approximately 80–85%, which would be optimum and of the most benefit to the patient. When using any airway adjunct it is very important after inhalation, to observe the patient's chest to ensure the rise and fall before administering the next breath. If it does

MEDICAL EMERGENCIES

not, reposition the mask to reduce any possible leakage and alter the position of the head to ensure that the patient has a patent airway.

The recovery position

The recovery position is also known as the lateral position. A patient is placed in this position when their circulation and breathing have been restored following an emergency. Placing a patient in the recovery position allows the tongue to fall forward keeping the airway clear. This is important so that the patient is provided with a patent airway and it also prevents the tongue from causing an obstruction, minimising the risk of gastric contents being inhaled [8].

The procedure

If the patient is not on their back you should carefully place them in this position with both their legs straight (Figure 6.23). Kneel beside the patient and remove anything bulky from their pockets, glasses if worn and turn any large rings around so that the bulky area is to their palm side. The patient's airway needs to be opened by a head tilt and chin lift action. The patient's arm that is nearest to you should be placed at right angles to their body so that the elbow is bent, with the palm of their hand being uppermost (Figure 6.24). With your left hand gently grasp their other hand (Figure 6.25), the one farthest away and bring it across their chest, holding it in place against their face on the cheek nearest to you (Figure 6.26). With your other hand grip the leg farthest away just above the knee and pull it up so that the foot is as flat

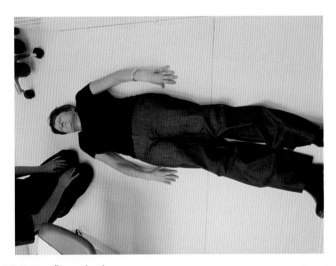

Figure 6.23 Patient flat on back.

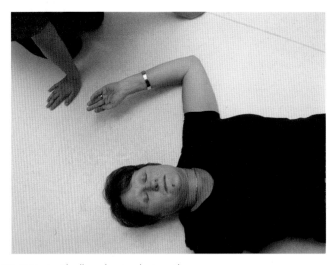

Figure 6.24 Patient with elbow bent palm to ceiling.

as possible on the ground (Figure 6.27). With gentle pressure keep their hand pressed against their cheek and pull on their leg so that the patient rolls towards you onto their side (Figure 6.28). When carrying this out very little resistance will be felt. There is no need to be forceful when rolling them. Once the patient is settled you should adjust the upper leg (the one you used to roll the patient over) so that both their hip and knee are bent at right angles (Figure 6.29). This action will provide a stable position for the patient. Finally, you must

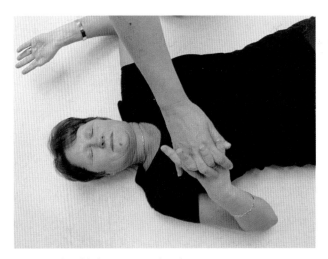

Figure 6.25 Rescuer's hand linking patient's hand.

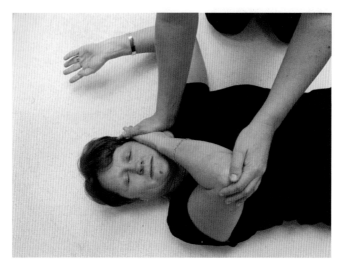

Figure 6.26 Rescuer holding patient's hand on their cheek.

ensure that the patient's airway has remained open by head tilting and chin lifting. You may have to adjust the hand under the patient's cheek to ensure this. Throughout this procedure you must provide constant reassurance to the patient, explaining each action as you carry it out and continually monitor the patient's breathing. Once placed in this position it is still very necessary to monitor the patient's vital signs watching for any sign of regression [8].

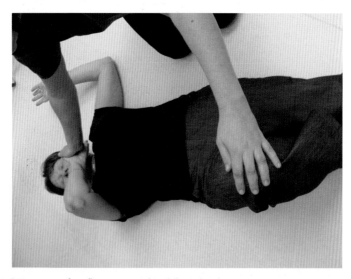

Figure 6.27 Patient's foot flat on ground with knee bent.

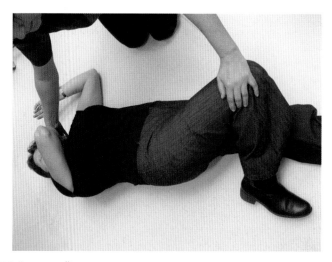

Figure 6.28 Rescuer rolling patient over.

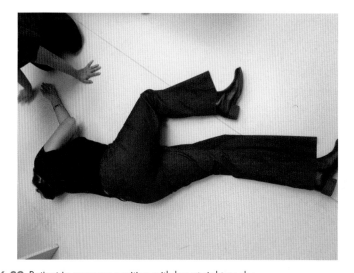

Figure 6.29 Patient in recovery position with leg at right angles.

BIBLIOGRAPHY

1. Resuscitation Council (U.K.), Medical emergencies and resuscitation. Standards for clinical practice and training for dental practitioners and dental care professionals in general dental practice, (July 2006; revised 2008).
2. http://www.nhlbi.nih.gov/health/dci/Diseases/Angina/Angina_WhatIs.html
3. http://www.epilepsysociety.org.uk/AboutEpilepsy
4. http://endocrine.niddk.nih.gov/pubs/addison/addison.htm

MEDICAL EMERGENCIES

5. http://www.nhlbi.nih.gov/health/dci/Diseases/Asthma/Asthma_WhatIs.html
6. http://www.nhlbi.nih.gov/health/dci/Diseases/HeartAttack/HeartAttack_WhatIs.html
7. http://www.nhlbi.nih.gov/health/dci/Diseases/scda/scda_whatis.html
8. Bristol Dental Hospital Course notes.
9. American Heart Association.

MEDICAL EMERGENCIES

Chapter 7

Essential anatomy

LEARNING OUTCOMES

At the end of this chapter you will have a clear understanding of:

- The heart, blood and the circulation of the blood through the heart, the respiratory system and their relevance to conscious sedation.
- The sites for venepuncture and associated veins.

INTRODUCTION

When undertaking conscious sedation, knowledge of specific anatomy is essential in order to understand how the various sedation techniques administered to patients act and work within their bodies. Increased awareness will aid identification of the potential complications, because the action of each is known.

THE BLOOD

The human blood is a fluid connective tissue which forms the transport system of the body. Without it the body would cease to function. An adult body contains approximately 5L of blood (8.80 pints), which accounts for approximately 7–8% of their total body weight. It has a pH of 7.4 and four main groups A, B, AB, and O, with O being the most common and the universal recipient from all other groups. Blood is made up of plasma, which equates to 55% of the volume and three types of blood cells – red, white and platelets, which make up the remaining 45% of the volume. Blood cells are sometimes

Basic Guide to Dental Sedation Nursing, First Edition. Nicola Rogers.
© 2011 Nicola Rogers. Published 2011 by Blackwell Publishing Ltd.

referred to as corpuscles, with all being produced in the bone marrow, which is a soft spongy material that fills the cavities of the bones. Every day millions of red and white blood cells are produced and formed by a healthy person [1–3].

Red corpuscles

They make up 99% of the total number of blood cells and are also known as erythrocytes. Their main function is to carry oxygen from the lungs to the cells within the body and help remove the waste carbon dioxide for transportation to the lungs to be exhaled. They perform this function through the haemoglobin, an iron containing protein to which the oxygen attaches, giving the blood its red colour. They are circular in shape and have a dip in the middle, making them bi-concave discs, which increases their surface area, thus allowing more oxygen to be carried to the cells of the body. Circulating red blood cells have a life span of approximately 120 days, with their membrane becoming fragile as they age. They cannot repair themselves, with many dying in the spleen. As they become trapped in the narrow channel they get broken and destroyed. During this process the haemoglobin is further broken down into its different components which are either recycled in the body or disposed of. A deficiency of haemoglobin is called anaemia [1,2].

White corpuscles

They are also known as leucocytes. Their main function is to help the body fight infections by circulating, awaiting transportation to an infected site. They are phagocytes, increasing in number when infections are present, to protect the body, by engulfing and destroying micro-organisms and removing dead or injured tissue. They are larger than the red blood cells, variable in shape with a nucleus, but fewer in number. Their life span is approximately 13–21 days. Leukaemia is a malignant disease affecting these cells [1,2].

Platelets

These are the smallest of the blood cells whose function is to assist clotting. They are also known as thrombocytes and are small, oval, colourless sticky discs that do not have a nucleus and are irregular in shape. Their life span is 8–10 days and without them bleeding would not be arrested. They circulate around the body, inactive until they meet a severed vessel whereupon they gather at the site of the injury and their sticky surface, coupled with other substances within the blood form a clot to block the flow. Unfortunately, they can form a clot even when a vessel has not been severed. This can lead to deep vein thrombosis which is dangerous as it can cut the flow to an area of the body and prevent entry of oxygenated blood. A stroke is a result of a clot that has lodged in an artery of the brain. If it is suspected that a patient has an abnormal clotting time then it can be investigated by providing a blood test known as 'International Normalised Ratio', which establishes their clotting time. Haemophilia, Von Willebrand's disease and Christmas disease are all very similar and all are caused by a missing factor in the coagulation of the blood [1, 2].

Plasma

This is the liquid element of the blood which is mainly formed from water. It is a clear, slightly alkaline, straw-coloured fluid which is used as a transport medium and carries blood cells and various other substances throughout the body, such as hormones, nutrients, proteins, iron, antibodies, clotting substances and waste products [1].

Blood composition

- 92% water.
- Nutrients – glucose from foods containing carbohydrates, amino acids from foods containing proteins and vitamins from all foods.
- Mineral salts – sodium chloride and bicarbonate, both of which help the blood to maintain its slight alkalinity.
- Waste products – mainly carbon dioxide and urea.
- Plasma proteins – albumen, which gives the blood its sticky texture.
- Clotting substances – prothrombin and fibrinogen.
- Antibodies – protein substances produced by the lymphatic system cells in response to the presence of an antigen to which it is antagonistic.
- Hormones – secretions from the endocrine glands [1].

Functions of blood

- To transport oxygen to the tissues via the haemoglobin within the red cells.
- To remove waste products from the tissues for transportation to the appropriate organs for excretion, for example:
  - Carbon dioxide is carried to the lungs to be exhaled.
  - Urea is carried from the liver to the kidneys to be excreted.
  - Water is carried to the kidneys, lungs and skin where any excess is removed.
- To transport nourishment to all parts of the body.
- To transport hormones, for example: insulin from the pancreas.
- To transport antibodies which fight infection.
- To aid defence of the body through the white blood cells.
- Distribute heat throughout the body and assist with temperature control.
- To coagulate and seal any cut blood vessel within the circulatory system [1].

ESSENTIAL ANATOMY

THE HEART

The human heart is approximately the same size as an individual's fist and requires oxygen to grow, because as an individual's body grows so does the heart. That is why a baby's heart rate is faster than a small childs, as their growth is more rapid. The heart receives the increased oxygen provided through the faster heart rate. As a person gets older the heart rate slows down and is generally stabilised by the age of 18, when the heart is fully developed (Figure 7.1). A heartbeat can be felt where an artery passes over a bone and is known as a pulse. This is a wave of distension of the artery which travels to the periphery and is referred to as beats per minute and will increase or decrease according to the requirement of the body. There are various areas around the body where a pulse can be felt, with the most common being the radial (Table 7.1). A blockage in any part or all of the vessels that supply the heart will cause a heart attack and if it is not cleared quickly will cause permanent damage to the heart muscle, reducing the effectiveness of the heart's pumping action. The heart should be looked after by leading a healthy life, hopefully preventing disease [1,4,5].

The heart is divided into four chambers. It has two upper chambers known as the atrium, one on the right and one on the left and two lower chambers known as the ventricles, one on the right and one on the left. The right side of the heart contains deoxygenated blood and the left side oxygenated blood. They are divided by a septum, which provides a dense muscle wall to prevent leakage (Figure 7.2). The amount of blood flow through the heart is controlled by valves, which also prevents the blood flowing backwards, ensuring a continuous flow through the heart. The heart is situated between the lungs and underneath the sternum (breast bone), to the left of the chest cavity. It acts as a double pump, pumping blood from the heart to the lungs to become oxygenated. This is known as pulmonary circulation. It also pumps oxygenated blood around

ESSENTIAL ANATOMY

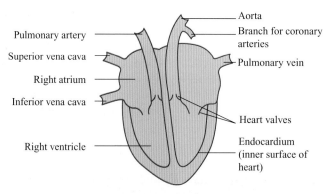

Figure 7.1 Diagram of the heart. (From Hollins, C. (2008) *Levison's Textbook for Dental Nurses*, 10th edn. Reproduced with permission from John Wiley & Sons.)

Table 7.1 Pulses situated around the body.

Pulse	Region of the body
Temporal	Ear
Facial	Chin
Carotid	Trachea
Brachial	Antecubital fossa
Ulnar	Baby finger side of wrist
Radial	Thumb side of wrist
Femoral	Groin region
Popliteal	Knee region
Posterior tibial	Ankle region
Dorsalis	Front of foot
Apical	Heart

the body, known as systemic circulation. The heart muscle receives oxygenated blood through coronary circulation [1].

Blood flow through the heart

The blood that has circulated around the body supplying it with oxygen and collecting the waste carbon dioxide returns to the heart without oxygen. It enters the heart via two vena cava vessels, with the superior vena cava receiving blood from the upper body and the inferior vena cava receiving blood from the lower part of the body. It then enters the right atrium and opens the tricuspid valve due to its weight, allowing the blood to enter the right ventricle. The tricuspid valve closes to prevent reverse flow. The right ventricle contracts to force the blood through the semilunar valve at the entrance to the pulmonary artery and is then transported to the lungs. An exchange of gases occurs (explained later on in this chapter). The oxygen-rich blood returns to the left side of the heart via the pulmonary veins (two from each lung) to enter the left atrium. Due to its weight, the blood opens the mitral valve (also known as the bicuspid valve) to enter the left ventricle. The mitral valve closes to prevent reverse flow. The left ventricle contracts to push the blood through the semilunar valve at the opening to the aorta where the heart muscle receives sufficient blood supply (Figure 7.3). The remainder is then circulated around the body to repeat the process. The right and left common carotid arteries supply the aorta with blood. They lie in the neck and divide into the right and left internal and

Right atrium	Septum	Left atrium
Right ventricle		Left ventricle

Figure 7.2 Diagram showing septum which divides the right and left sides of the heart.

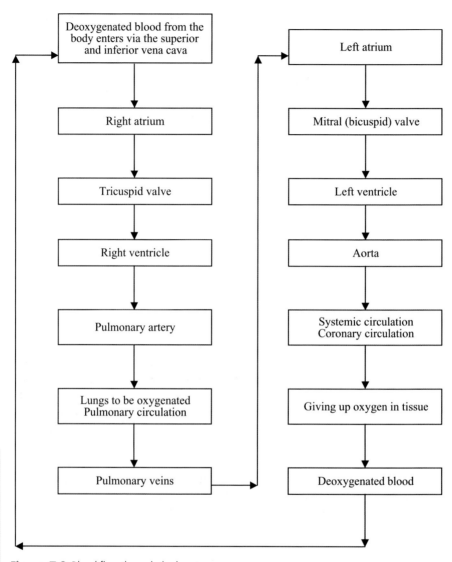

Figure 7.3 Blood flow through the heart.

external carotid arteries, with the internal artery supplying blood to the skull and brain and the external artery to the face and scalp [1].

THE RESPIRATORY SYSTEM

The respiratory system's function is to supply the blood with oxygen for transportation to all parts of the body. This takes place through breathing.

ESSENTIAL ANATOMY

Our cells require energy and it is largely obtained as a result of chemical reactions. These reactions can take place only in the presence of oxygen, with the main waste product being carbon dioxide. Oxygen is necessary for life and when in combustion with food it produces energy for all the cells. Therefore the respiratory system provides a route for oxygen, present in the atmospheric air, to enter the body when we breathe in and an exit for carbon dioxide to be expelled when we breathe out. Inhaled atmospheric air consists of approximately:

- 79% nitrogen
- 20% oxygen
- 1.0% trace gases of which 0.04% is carbon dioxide

Of the 20% oxygen inhaled, the body only uses 4% as it is exchanged for 4% carbon dioxide. We then exhale 16% oxygen and 4.04% carbon dioxide [1,6,7].

Respiration

There are two types of respiration – external and internal.

External respiration is when the gases in the atmospheric air exchange with those present in the lungs (Figure 7.4). Internal respiration is when the gases in the blood exchange with those present in the tissue cells (Figure 7.5). The passage through which the atmospheric air reaches the lungs is known as the respiratory tract. It is divided into an upper and lower respiratory tract. The upper tract comprises the nose, the nasal cavity, the pharynx and the larynx, whereas the lower tract comprises the trachea, bronchi and the lungs. The chest cavity is separated from the abdominal cavity by the diaphragm and all air passages are lined with columnar epithelium cells [1].

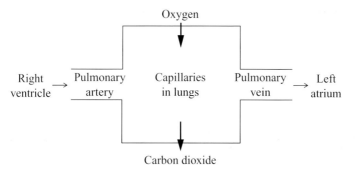

Figure 7.4 External respiration. (From Hollins, C. (2008) *Levison's Textbook for Dental Nurses*, 10th edn. Reproduced with permission from John Wiley & Sons.)

ESSENTIAL ANATOMY

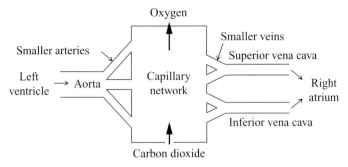

Figure 7.5 Internal respiration. (From Hollins, C. (2008) *Levison's Textbook for Dental Nurses*, 10th edn. Reproduced with permission from John Wiley & Sons.)

Structures of the respiratory system and the passage of air (Figures 7.6 and 7.7)

The nose and nasal cavity

The nose is divided into two chambers, separated by a nasal septum. The central portion of the nose is lined with cilia, which are hair-like substances. These cilia protect the air passages as they prevent any foreign material, such

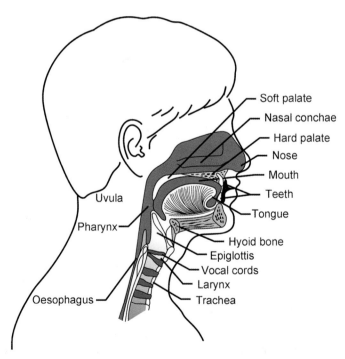

Figure 7.6 Upper airway. (From Girdler, N., Hill, C. and Wilson, K. (2009) *Clinical Sedation in Dentistry*. Reproduced with permission from John Wiley & Sons.)

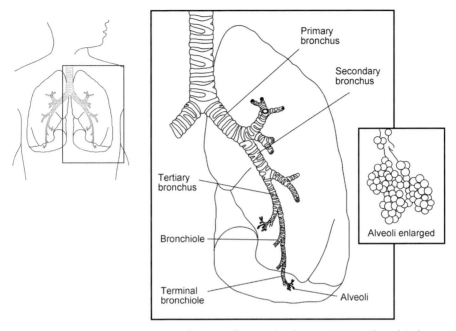

Figure 7.7 Lower airway. (From Girdler, N., Hill, C. and Wilson, K. (2009) *Clinical Sedation in Dentistry*. Reproduced with permission from John Wiley & Sons.)

as dirt, dust or mucous, from entering the nose. The cilia collect any foreign body/bodies, causing them to be blown or sneezed away from the nose. As air enters the nasal passages it is warmed and moistened as it makes contact with the moist mucus within the nose. It is also filtered so that any dust or other foreign bodies stick to the mucus, with the cilia of the mucous membrane wafting the mucus towards the throat to be swallowed.

The pharynx

The pharynx is also known as the throat. It is a muscular tube, approximately 5 inches long, situated behind the nose, the mouth and the larynx, connecting the nose (nasopharynx), the mouth (oropharynx) and the larynx (laryngopharynx). Once the air leaves the nose it enters the nasopharynx to travel to the oropharynx (Figure 7.8) and then into the laryngopharynx. The air continues to be moistened, warmed and filtered. The mouth not only allows air to be breathed in but also provides a route for food to enter our bodies. Once the food has been masticated, it passes from the mouth, through the oropharynx, into the oesophagus. When food is swallowed the epiglottis closes over the inlet to the larynx to direct the food into the oesophagus, blocking the entrance to the trachea and prevents entry to the respiratory tract. If any food went down the wrong way chocking would occur. As a natural reflex coughing would ensue in an attempt to dislodge the offending food. It is important to ensure

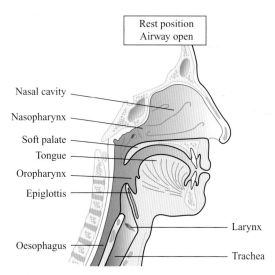

Figure 7.8 Section of the respiratory system showing the nasopharynx and the oropharynx. (From Hollins, C. (2008) *Levison's Textbook for Dental Nurses*, 10th edn. Reproduced with permission from John Wiley & Sons.)

that excellent aspiration is provided when patients are receiving treatment, keeping the pharynx free of secretions. When sedation is provided a patient's reflexes remain intact, which is one of the safety features of the technique, so there is no need to deny them food and drink. However, some clinicians prefer their patients to be starved, whereas others ask them to have a light snack a few hours before the procedure. With a general anaesthetic it is mandatory for a patient to be starved of food for 6 hours prior to the procedure, because the anaesthetic removes the patient's natural reflexes of swallowing or choking. By ensuring that the stomach is empty there is no danger of regurgitation into the oesophagus and inhalation into the lungs [1].

The larynx

The larynx is sometimes referred to as the 'Adam's Apple'. It is made up of several cartilages and sits on top of the trachea at the upper end. It contains the vocal cords within the thyroid cartilage which can be seen to move on swallowing. In adult males, it is larger, allowing longer vocal cords which give a deeper voice. The volume of a person's voice depends upon the amount of air that is forced past the vocal cords, with the quality of their voice being dependent upon the position of the tongue, the shape of their mouth and their sinuses. If it becomes inflamed a person would suffer laryngitis and their voice would sound very hoarse. The larynx withstands differences in air pressures and remains open to allow inhalation and exhalation at the same time. It is the main organ that initiates the cough reflex and will send any mucus upwards to the pharynx to be swallowed. As previously explained it is protected by

ESSENTIAL ANATOMY

the epiglottis and is made up of cartilage, ensuring that the airway remains open, preventing collapse. The first section of cartilage is known as the cricoid, which is connected to the thyroid by a thin membrane. If a laryngeal blockage occurred and it was impossible to ventilate the patient by other means then an emergency procedure, known as a cricothyrotomy, would be undertaken by making an incision through the skin and cricothyroid membrane to secure a patent airway. This enables the patient to breathe [1].

The trachea and the bronchial tree

The trachea is lined with mucus membrane and cilia which waft any foreign bodies up into the pharynx to be either coughed up or swallowed. It is approximately 12cm long and made up of incomplete rings of cartilage which are connected by fibrous tissues. The cartilage rings are incomplete at the back of the trachea to allow the oesophagus to expand and contract during swallowing. The base of the trachea then divides into two branches known as primary bronchi, one to the right lung and the other to the left. If an item is dropped to the back of the pharynx to enter the respiratory tract it is more likely to fall into the right bronchi as the branch is more vertical than the left and is slightly higher and shorter. The diaphragm is also slightly higher on the right. These primary bronchi then sub-divide into secondary and tertiary bronchi which then branch further into smaller tubes known as bronchioles and terminate in air sacs known as alveoli. These are lined with a delicate layer of flattened epithelial cells, which are surrounded by numerous capillaries. It is through these capillaries and flattened epithelial cells that the interchange of gases takes place. The blood in the capillaries is transported to the lungs through the pulmonary artery and is deoxygenated. Once the exchange of carbon dioxide and oxygen takes place, the blood, now oxygenated, is transported to the left side of the heart through the pulmonary veins and is circulated around the body [1].

The lungs and the pleura

There are two lungs, one on the left side and the other on the right, which, together with the heart, occupy the entire chest cavity. As the diaphragm is higher on the right the right lung is shorter. The left lung is slightly smaller and lighter than the right due to the heart sitting on the left side of the pleural cavity. Each lung is divided into lobes, with the right having three (superior, middle and inferior) lobes and the left having two (superior and inferior) (Figure 7.9). These lobes divide further into lobules, which are pyramidal in shape [1].

Pleura comprises of two layers of slippery membranes – an inner and outer layer which surround the lungs, allowing expansion and contraction and holding them against the chest wall to avoid collapse. The lungs will collapse because of a pneumothorax. Inflammation of the pleura is called pleurisy, where pain is

ESSENTIAL ANATOMY

Right lung	Left lung
Superior	Superior
Middle	Inferior
Inferior	

Figure 7.9 Diagram showing lung division.

felt after a deep breath has been taken. This is due to the pleura being stretched and friction between the inflamed surfaces [1].

The diaphragm and the intercostal muscles

The diaphragm separates the chest cavity from the abdominal cavity. It is a strong muscular partition that moves up and down like a piston to enlarge the chest area every time it descends. When a person inhales the diaphragm and the intercostal muscles that are situated between each rib contract, increasing the size of the thorax by raising the ribs upwards and outwards, allowing atmospheric air to enter the lungs. To accommodate air the lungs increase in size. When a person exhales the lungs return to their normal size, allowing the air to expel as the diaphragm and intercostal muscles relax and return to their normal position. The process of the diaphragm contracting allows the oxygen to be pulled into the lungs and when it relaxes, it allows the carbon dioxide to be pumped out of the lungs [1].

The process of respiration

Respiration is controlled by the brain and the frequency of breathing is directly related to the amount of carbon dioxide in the blood. When the levels are elevated a breath is taken to remove the waste carbon dioxide from the body. This action is normally involuntary but can be altered by a voluntary action and emotional control (i.e. holding of breath or sobbing). If breathing stops for any reason then the carbon dioxide level increases and results in the sensors within the body sending a message to the respiratory centre within the brain to make the breathing deeper and faster. This eliminates the increased carbon dioxide and breathing should be restored to normal. Exercise will increase the rate and depth of respiration, as the oxygen is used by the cells more quickly, producing carbon dioxide at a faster rate than normal. To eliminate it, breathing becomes faster. Breathing occurs when the lungs expand to take in the atmospheric air and then contract to expel it. This occurs because of muscular activity which is partly voluntary and partly involuntary. During normal breathing, the muscles in action are the intercostal muscles and the diaphragm. If difficulties are experienced when breathing they are aided by

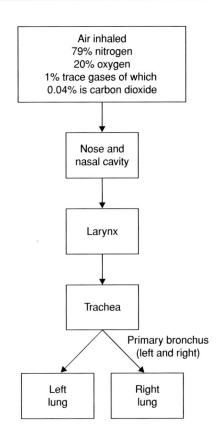

Figure 7.10 Diagram showing passage of air through the respiratory tract.

the muscles of the abdomen, the neck and the shoulders. When monitoring respiration, there are three phases to a cycle: (1) inspiration, (2) expiration and (3) a pause before the next cycle. Respiration is achieved through the respiratory tract, with the atmospheric air passing through each structure until it reaches the lungs where the gaseous exchange takes place (Figure 7.10). It enters the respiratory system through the mouth and nose, through the larynx, into the trachea and into the left and right bronchi to the bronchial tubes which connect to the tiny alveoli sacs [1].

Adult lungs contain approximately 600 million air-filled sacs which are surrounded by capillaries. The inhaled oxygen within the atmospheric air passes into the alveoli and then diffuses through the capillaries into the arterial deoxygenated blood. At the same time, the deoxygenated, waste-rich blood, containing carbon dioxide from the veins releases the carbon dioxide into the alveoli to be exhaled via the same route. This exchange of oxygen for carbon dioxide occurs by diffusion across the alveolar capillary membrane, with the rate and direction dependent upon the partial pressure that each gas exerts. Inhaled air within the lungs contains a higher partial pressure of oxygen than the blood (20%) – consequently, the oxygen diffuses from the alveoli air

ESSENTIAL ANATOMY

(a) Oxygen

Oxygen in the lungs	Oxygen in the blood	Concentration of oxygen diffused across the alveoli air sacs	Concentration of oxygen exhaled
20%	None	4%	16%

(b) Carbon dioxide

Carbon dioxide in the lungs	Carbon dioxide in the blood	Concentration of carbon dioxide exhaled
0.04%	High	4.04%

Figure 7.11 Diagram showing exchange of gases.

sacs into the blood. The reverse occurs with the carbon dioxide, as the air within the lungs contains a lower partial pressure of carbon dioxide (0.04%) than that in the blood. The carbon dioxide leaves the blood, diffusing into the alveolar air sacs in the lungs. There is an exchange of 4% oxygen for 4% carbon dioxide (Figure 7.11). This means that the blood now contains oxygen which is transported to the left side of the heart via the pulmonary veins and the lungs are in receipt of carbon dioxide which will be exhaled as waste gas through the respiratory tract [1].

This process occurs because gases diffuse from a higher to a lower concentration/percentage. They are always in motion and will exert pressure on the container they are held in and if there is a hole they will escape. The atmospheric air entering the lungs also contains nitrogen, inert gases and water vapour. These, coupled with oxygen and carbon dioxide, exert pressure on the walls of the alveoli equal to that of the atmospheric pressure. Each gas has a partial pressure and together they make up the total pressure, with each being proportional to its concentration. As the partial pressure of nitrogen is the same in both the alveoli and the blood it remains stable, because nitrogen, as a gas, is not used by the body – however, it can diffuse across the walls of the alveoli and the capillaries. The pressure of gases within the blood, when leaving the lungs via the pulmonary veins, remains the same as the alveoli air. As the blood moves slowly through the capillaries surrounding the alveoli it allows time for the interchange of gases to take place and for oxygen to be taken by the erythrocytes in the blood. The oxygen is dissolved in the plasma and combines with the haemoglobin to produce oxyhaemoglobin, which, as an unstable compound, breaks up easily to release the oxygen. The process of internal respiration is exactly the same as external in that the diffusion of gases occurs from the higher to the lower concentration/percentage. In this instance the concentration of oxygen in the blood exceeds that of the vital organs and cells. The cells then receive oxygen. At the same time carbon dioxide is diffused into the blood as a waste product of carbohydrate and fat metabolism of the cells, because the concentration/percentage of carbon dioxide is higher in the vital organs and cells than that of the blood. This process is continuous as the cells require a constant supply of oxygen and is based on supply and demand. This means that if activity is increased in an area within the body the cells will receive more oxygen reflecting those changes because the carbon dioxide will be higher as a result of the altered activity. Areas where activity is either normal or reduced will only receive oxygen proportional to their need. Some patients, due to fear, may increase their breathing voluntarily, which will result in the carbon dioxide within the blood being reduced. This in turn results in their breathing stopping for a while, because breathing is reliant on the level of carbon dioxide being raised. This condition is known as hyperventilation, which could develop into tetany, where their muscles contract and go into spasms. To treat this condition patients should be calmed and reassured in an attempt to control their breathing. They should be requested to breathe in and out of a paper bag in order that they re-breathe their carbon dioxide, as the contents of the bag will contain expired air. By re-breathing their own carbon dioxide breathing should be restored to normal. Under no circumstance should oxygen be given as this treatment works in the same way as respiration, because gases will go from the higher to the lower concentration/percentage [1].

THE DORSUM OF THE HAND AND THE ANTECUBITAL FOSSA

For intravenous sedation to be provided the clinician will place and secure a cannula into the patient's vein in order to administer the drug/s and to provide continuous venous access for the administration of emergency drug/s should the need arise. The sites commonly used for venepuncture are the antecubital fossa and the dorsum of the hand. The clinician will, of course, understand the anatomical structure of both sites allowing safe insertion of their preferred cannula. There are advantages and disadvantages (Table 7.2) of using both areas to cannulate a patient, so the selected site is dependent upon the preference of the clinician, coupled with identifying a suitable vein (Figures 7.12a and b) [1].

The dorsum of the hand

It is also known as the back of the hand. It is thought that as it is difficult for a patient to bend their hand back that this area provides a relatively safe place to

Table 7.2 Advantages and disadvantages of cannulation sites.

Cannulation site	Advantages	Disadvantages
Antecubital fossa	Larger veins If bruising occurs, it can be hidden under clothing	Depending upon the cannula used the arm may need stabilising to restrict movement, therefore avoiding damage to deeper anatomical structures Accidental injection into the brachial artery or aberrant ulnar artery
Dorsum of the hand	Easy access	If bruising occurs, it can be painful and is more obvious

insert and secure a cannula. The veins (known as the dorsal venous network) which drain from the cephalic and basilic veins on the dorsum of the hand are immediately under the skin so there are no deeper anatomical structures to cause concern (Figure 7.13) [1].

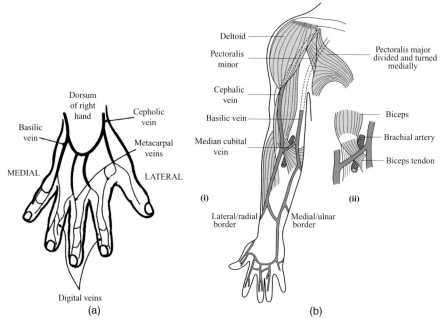

Figure 7.12 (a) Dorsum of the hand. (From Ireland, R.S. (2010) *Advanced Dental Nursing*, 2nd edn. Reproduced with permission from John Wiley & Sons. Original source: Girdler, N. and Hill, C. (1998) *Clinical Sedation in Dentistry*.) (b) Venous anatomy of the arm. (From Ireland, R.S. (2010) *Advanced Dental Nursing*, 2nd edn. Reproduced with permission from John Wiley & Sons. Original source: Ellis, H. (2002) *Clinical Anatomy*, 12th edn.)

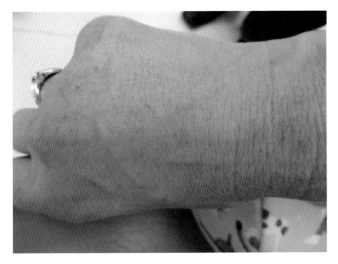

Figure 7.13 Dorsum of the hand.

The antecubital fossa

This is the area of the arm located at the inner aspect of the elbow. The basilic vein, found on the medial aspect of the arm (baby finger side), and the cephalic vein supply this area and both are commonly used. There are a number of veins connecting them, the main one being the median basilic. As the brachial artery lies in this area the clinician will insert a cannula superficially in order to avoid it and other deeper anatomical structures (Figure 7.14). It must be remembered that if a butterfly needle is the clinician's preferred choice, the patient's arm

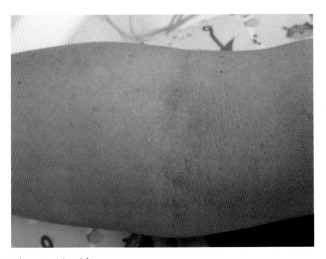

Figure 7.14 The antecubital fossa.

ESSENTIAL ANATOMY

must be stabilised using an arm board to prevent movement. This avoids the needle being forced out of the vein and further into that area. Stabilisation of the arm is not required with a Venflon as the indwelling cannula is made of pliable plastic and will not cause damage if the patient does move his/her arm [1].

BIBLIOGRAPHY

1. Bristol Dental Hospital course notes.
2. www.homehealth-uk.com/medical/blood.htm
3. www.virtualmedicalcentre.com/?centre=blo
4. en.wikepedia.org/wiki/Heart
5. ww.fi.edu/learn/heart/
6. en.wikepedia.org/wiki/Respiratory System
7. www.virtualmedicalcentre.com/anatomy.asp?sid=16

ESSENTIAL ANATOMY

Index

Note: Page numbers with italicised *f*'s and *t*'s refer to figures and tables, respectively.